The Roseto Story

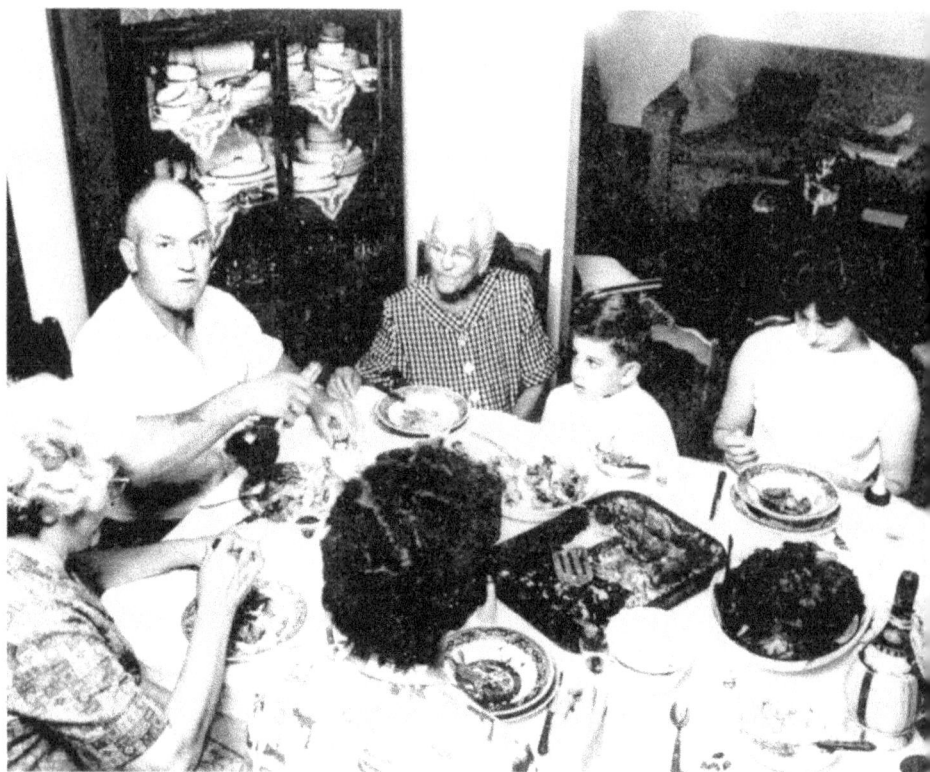

A Roseto family at table, 1964.

THE ROSETO STORY

An Anatomy of Health

by
John G. Bruhn and Stewart Wolf
Photographs by Remsen Wolff

Norman
University of Oklahoma Press

Library of Congress Cataloging in Publication Data

Bruhn, John G
The Roseto Story.

Bibliography: p.
Includes index.
1. Heart — Pennsylvania — Roseto — Mortality.
2. Italian Americans — Social life and customs. 4. Health
surveys — Pennsylvania — Roseto. 5. Roseto, Pa. — Social
conditions. 6. Coronary heart disease — Social aspects. I.
Wolf, Stewart George, 1914– joint author. II. Title.
RA645.H4B78   616.1'23'071   78-21364
ISBN 978-0-8061-3613-8 (paper)

Dedicated to Mark R. Everett, Dean of Medicine, University of Oklahoma Health Sciences Center, 1947 to 1966, and George L. Cross, President of the University of Oklahoma, 1944 to 1968, whose commitment to scholarship afforded permission and encouragement for this extensive off-campus research

Preface

Roseto, an Italian-American community in North-ampton County, east-central Pennsylvania, provides striking evidence of a correlation between health, especially cardiovascular and mental health, and the character of human relationships in a community. Roseto, an ethnic enclave settled nearly a century ago, enjoyed a remarkably low death rate from heart attack (myocardial infarction) and a low incidence of mental illness, especially senile dementia.

Our study was prompted by the observation of a physician, Dr. Benjamin Falcone, that myocardial infarction was relatively uncommon among Rosetans. Dr. Falcone, who had practiced medicine for seventeen years in the vicinity, had noted the rarity of heart attacks among Rosetans in their forties and fifties, while the rate of heart attacks in men of comparable age in the United States was increasing. We were able to confirm Dr. Falcone's observations by a careful study of health records and learned that the death rate for all ages in Roseto from myocardial infarction was 1 per thousand males and 0.6 per thousand females, a very low rate compared to the average in the United States of 3.5 per thousand males and 2.09 per thousand females. We found that death rates from myocardial infarction in two neighboring towns, Bangor and Nazareth, matched the mean for the nation. Moreover, those dying from myocardial infarction in the neighboring communities included many Italians, some of them relatives of Rosetans, and even individuals born in Roseto who had moved away at an early age with their parents.

We and several of our colleagues from the University of Oklahoma then undertook to compare medical histories, physical examinations, and laboratory tests on a large sample of Rosetans and inhabitants of the two neighboring communities. We found a striking absence of the stigmata of coronary heart disease among Rosetans relative to their neighbors. The findings were surprising because of a greater prevalence of obesity among Rosetans. A meticulous study of dietary habits established that Rosetans ate at least as much animal fat as did the inhabitants of Bangor and Nazareth. The prevalence of hypertension and diabetes and measures of serum cholesterol concentration were closely similar in all three communities. We also found that smoking and exercise habits in the three towns differed little.

Thus it appeared that an absence of conventionally accepted "risk factors" for coronary heart disease could not explain the Rosetans' relative immunity from fatal heart attacks. We were also able to rule out ethnic and genetic factors as an explanation for the differences observed. One striking feature did set Roseto apart from its neighbors, however, namely its culture, which reflected tenaciously held Old World values and customs. We found that family relationships were extremely close and mutually supportive. This cohesive quality extended to neighbors and to the community as a whole. There was a well-defined man-woman relationship in Roseto, where the man was uncontested head of the family. The elderly were cherished and respected, and they retained their authority throughout life. The atmosphere of Roseto was gay and friendly and reflected an enthusiastic and optimistic attitude toward life. This book proposes the theory that the Rosetan way of life, its social pattern, may have contributed substantially to the healthy state of the community. Significantly, as traditional values are gradually being abandoned by the rising generation, the death rate from heart attack in Roseto appears to be climbing toward the American norm.

The research was supported by PHS Grant HE-06286-08 from the National Heart Institute and PHS

Grant MH-20400-01 from the National Institute of Mental Health. The work was begun when we were members of the faculty of the University of Oklahoma Health Sciences Center. Several colleagues from the Departments of Medicine, Preventive Medicine and Public Health, and Psychiatry and Behavioral Sciences participated in the studies including Drs. C. A. Adsett, Kurt Dubowski, Marshall E. Groover, C. G. Gunn, James Hampton, Paul Houk, T. N. Lynn, Richard Marshall, John Naughton, G. V. Rohrer, R. A. Schneider, John Scott, L. Clark Stout, and Johann Wulff. Lucille Boone, Cecilia Coffey, and Emogene Ogle, of the Department of Dietetics, and their students and several medical students and technicians in other departments made contributions to the study.

The following medical students and graduate students in sociology helped in the collection and analysis of sociological data: John T. Patterson, Asoke K. Basu, David Reynolds, Guy Danielson III, Fred Pumpian-Mindlin, Kaye Middleton Fillmore, Andrea and Gorst duPlessis, Gary Shapiro, E. N. Samara, Donald Barnett, Robert Krasnow, Peter Frank, Michael Smith, John George, A. R. Spalding III, Henry B. Bird, Billy U. Philips, Betty C. Chandler, Robert Bowser, Jim Goldsberry, and Kay'da Grace. Mrs. James H. Ross played a major role in organizing and coordinating the study.

Staff members of the Biostatistical Unit of the University of Oklahoma Health Sciences Center worked many hours assisting us with the analysis of data: Dr.

M. Clinton Miller, Dr. Albert Dorr, Dr. John McCoy, Dr. Vernon Ribera, and Paul Costiloe. Dr. Edward N. Brandt served as statistical consultant. Members of the Division of Data Processing and Biostatistics of the Pennsylvania Department of Health, especially Dr. Albert E. Bailey, George E. Greenwood, William R. Dixon, and H. Barrett Bock, were helpful in our study of death certificates and provided census and other data.

We are especially grateful to those physicians in Northampton County who helped at various stages of our study: Drs. James E. Brackbill, Thomas M. Carlyle, Francis J. Cinelli, Benjamin Falcone, Joseph L. Farace, George M. Gruver, J. Z. Heberling, Floyd M. Hess, Wesley Stancombe, Anthony Turtzo, and Stanley J. Walczyk. The generous assistance of Dr. Nicholas M. Romano, himself a Rosetan, was particularly valuable throughout the period of follow-up.

In addition to the photographs made by Remsen N. Wolff, we are grateful to Steve Schapiro and to Black Star Publishing Company, Inc., of New York, for permission to include their photographs.

Our research could not have been carried out without the permission and support of the Roseto Town Council, and we are indebted to the members of the council and to Mayors George Giaquinto and Charles C. Angelini. Special acknowledgment is due Florence Giaquinto, who served as coordinator of the study and was responsible for helping establish the excellent rapport that existed between the community and the research team throughout the study. Florence Giaquinto's sisters, Mary Carrescia, Virginia Donatelli, and Rose Cistone, as well as Dorothy Ruggiero and other Rosetans too many to cite, assisted in various ways over the years. Generous assistance in organizing the survey in Bangor was provided by Mrs. Sandy Peiffly Capone, and in Nazareth by Mrs. Harriet Frack.

The people of Roseto and their neighbors in Bangor and Nazareth provided the data and through their wholehearted cooperation and generous hospitality made this study possible.

For help in the preparation of the manuscript we are grateful to Helen Goodell, Joan Martin, Colleen Nagel, Cindy Carter, Susan Stevenson, and Moira Martin.

John G. Bruhn, PH.D.
Galveston, Texas

Stewart Wolf, M.D.
Bethlehem, Pennsylvania

Contents

Illustrations

The Roseto Story

1
Roseto in Historical Perspective

Cose e' l'America? Un massettino di fiori.
(What is America? A bunch of flowers.)
From a popular song in southern Italy in the 1880's.

In the 1800's southern Italy was in the throes of emigration fever, and some of the small villages were literally decimated. The landowners maintained a feudal hold over the villagers and tried to oppose emigration, but with little success. By the turn of the century approximately half a million southern Italians had traded their poverty for the uncertainty of America and settled mainly in the mid-Atlantic region—New York, New Jersey, and Pennsylvania (17, 44, 46).

One community eager to supply emigrants to the United States was Roseto Valfortore, a village of twenty-five hundred on the Adriatic side of southern Italy in the province of Foggia. The town is perched on a steeply slanting hillside near the top of a small

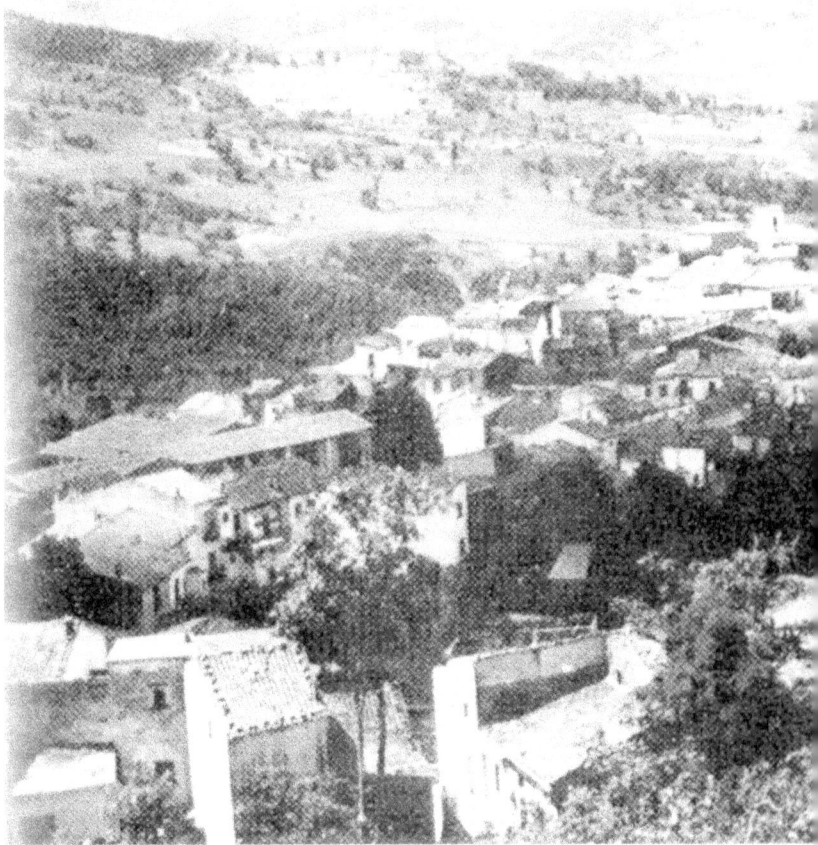

Roseto Valfortore in the province of Foggia in southern Italy.

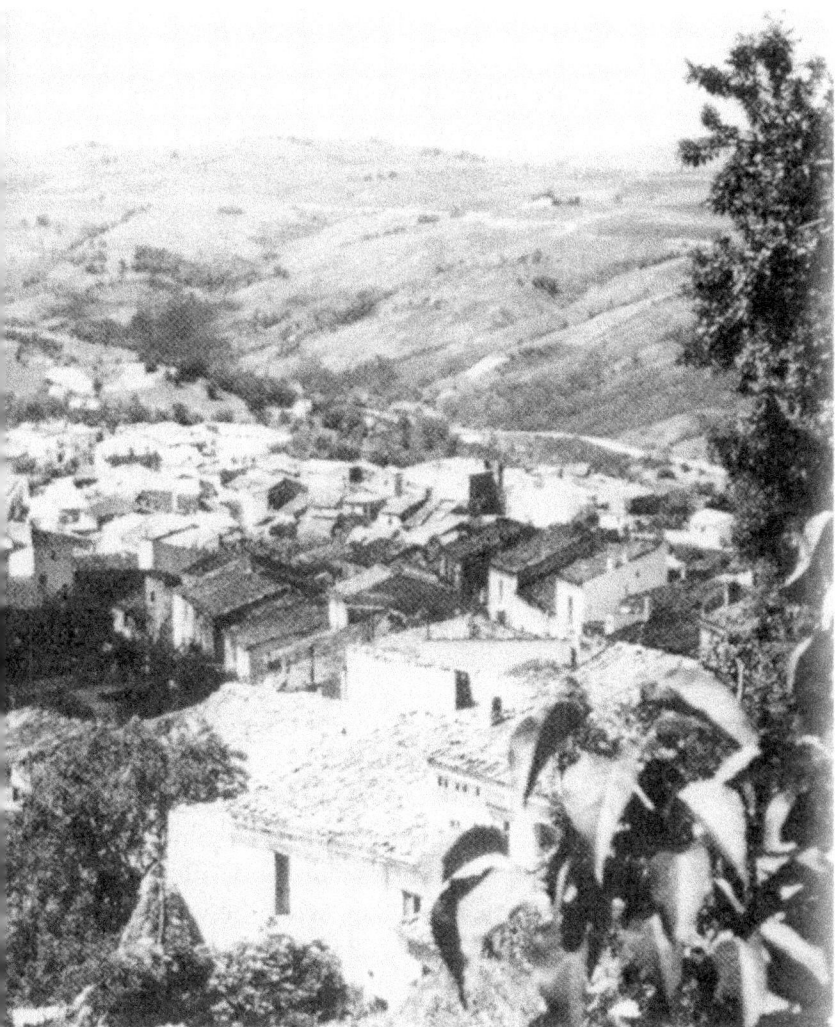

mountain that rises abruptly from the coastal plain. The maximum elevation is 1,150 meters, but the center of town is only 650 meters above sea level. Roseto Valfortore is near the border of neighboring Benevento Province, approximately thirty miles inland from the Adriatic seaport Bari. During the Roman era its rose-covered countryside prompted the name Rosetum. The way of life of the *paesani,* or villagers, has hardly changed over the past hundred years (3, 16). They farm small patches of rough ground on the terraced hillside and each year raise one or two pigs. The village, like half a dozen others scattered over the sides of the small mountain, is under the prefecture of Naples.

Most of southern Italy was in the grip of poverty toward the end of the last century, and the villagers were especially receptive to the tales of riches and the "good life" in America. By 1882 the first wave of emigrants from Roseto had sailed to New York, encouraged by enthusiastic letters written by a Jesuit priest from Baltimore, Luigi Sabetti. Father Sabetti, a native of Roseto, was the posthumous son and fifteenth child of the town's doctor. In 1849, when he was ten years old, his mother died. Unwilling to be a financial burden to his older siblings, the young boy determined to become a Jesuit priest. After schooling in Naples and in France, he was ordained to the priesthood in 1868. Three years later he sailed for the United States, where he joined Woodstock College in Maryland as professor of moral theology.

United States immigration laws at that time were nonrestrictive, and the passage to America was relatively inexpensive. The Italian authorities, however, considered emigration unpatriotic and at first declined permission to the Rosetans and a few other would-be emigrants from the nearby villages Biccari, Castelluccio Valmaggiore, and Alberona (28). After the local authorities finally relented, thanks to the persuasive efforts of several influential people, the first group of eleven Rosetans, ten men and one boy (joined by three men and one boy from Castelfranco) left Italy in January 1882 for New York (2). One of the steamer's passengers died from an infectious disease during the voyage, causing everyone to be quarantined for one month (4). When the passengers were finally allowed to disembark, the Rosetan travelers went directly to the Italian settlement on Mulberry Street, where they spent the night on a tavern floor. An Italian railroad contractor, exacting a commission of one dollar from each of them, promised them work at Perth Amboy, New Jersey. The offer turned out to be a swindle, but eventually they obtained employment through a New York City employment agency: three as carpenters in Polatka, Florida, and eight as slate-quarry laborers in Howell Town, Pennsylvania, now part of Bangor. The work in the quarry pits was not only strenuous and dangerous but also foreign to their experience as farmers and artisans. Consequently three of the Rosetans went off to other communities in the United States, and the fourth, Guiseppe

Albanese, homesick, returned to Italy, where he received a triumphant welcome. Despite his return home, he later became an active promoter of emigration (2).

Among those whom Albanese influenced was Guiseppe Cardo, a wealthy physician in his seventies. Declaring jokingly that the trip would rejuvenate him, Dr. Cardo sailed for America in 1883 with a group of fifteen needy peasants to whom he loaned travel money. He secured employment for them as laborers in Amsterdam, New York. After two months there, and an additional six months working on the railroad at Indian Springs, near Peterborough, Ontario, winter came, their jobs ended, and the group disbanded. They failed to repay Dr. Cardo who returned to Italy feeling deserted and embittered.

Several members of the disbanded group managed to reach Howell Town on the invitation of fellow Rosetans who had settled there the previous year. Employed as slate quarriers, they worked ten-hour shifts for about eight cents an hour and lived in one-room shacks that looked out on heaps of slate rubble. Unable to speak English, and tenaciously holding to Old World customs and habits, the Italians were shunned and treated as inferiors by the English and Welsh. Nevertheless, their competition as laborers was feared. Furthermore, after several knifing incidents involving a few young Sicilians living in the area, the Rosetans were required to observe a curfew. Despite these hardships, they worked conscientiously, scrupulously saving their money so that they might send to Italy for their relatives (2).

By 1894 the number of passports issued to Rosetans bound for America had reached 1,200, not including women and children and others who had left clandestinely. Local Italian authorities were helpless to stop such a mass emigration. They hesitated to impose restrictions for fear the villagers might rebel. Many who remained in Italy were able, with money sent by their relatives in America, to buy their homes and fields from their landlords, who were willing to sell because they feared that there would not be enough Rosetans left to work the land. Other Rosetans shuttled between Italy and America, trying to increase their earnings and property. For them expatriation was only a temporary expedient. Later, however, the requirements of the Immigration Act of 1917 and the quota system established by the acts of 1921 and 1924 encouraged many Italian Rosetans to make Pennsylvania their permanent home (31).

As the Italian population grew and prospered economically, the social restrictions imposed by the English and Welsh prompted them to build their own community, and in social isolation they achieved a remarkable degree of self-sufficiency. They selected a hillside tract that was linked to adjacent Bangor only by a rough wagon road and the tracks of the Central Railroad of New Jersey, which crossed it from north to south. The land could be bought cheaply and with little formality because it had been stripped of its trees, which had been sold for lumber. The sawmill had left it covered with rubbish, stumps, and stones. In this unpromising spot the Italians in 1887 founded their new town, calling it New Italy (34). The first house, which faced the railroad tracks, was built in 1888 by Nicola Rosato. Shortly thereafter Lorenzo Falcone constructed a shed finished in clapboards that would house fourteen people. He divided his land into lots and sold it to relatives and friends, thereby establishing the community New Italy (2).

Further building development continued during the years 1889 to 1892 as new immigrants arrived. Paths were widened to lanes, lots were fenced in, and additional houses were built as land purchases continued. As described by Valletta, immigrants ingeniously used available materials: native stone for building, slate for roofs, walls, and walks (42). They helped each other dig out and build stone foundations for houses that were at first four-room one-story stone structures. There were no privately owned stores at first, for the quarry workers were required to trade at company stores. There were no factories, no churches, and no druggists or doctors nearer than Bangor (13). In 1892 the New Italy Hotel was opened by the first naturalized citizen, Lorenzo Pacifico. He sold wine, beer, and liquor in addition to tickets for transoceanic trips. The travel money was handled through an Italian bank in New York City. Grocery stores and other shops soon opened in Roseto.

The Italians provided their own social life through the Mutual Aid Society of Saint Philip Neri, organized in 1895. Its main functions were to teach Americanism, parliamentary procedure, and religion. The Cornet Band, also organized in 1895, played on festive occasions such as the religious festival of Our Lady of Mount Carmel, held annually during the last week of July from 1884. Masses at the first Mount Carmel celebrations were said by priests from Philadelphia and New York City. During the years 1891 to 1894 the celebration took on a secular character, because there was no Italian priest available who could serve full time at the church. The festival attracted crowds of people, both Italian and American, from surrounding towns. Two brass bands, the Roma Band of Philadelphia and the Bersaglieri Band of New York City, played classical Italian music. In 1895 the festival featured the blessing of the American and Italian flags by an Italian priest from New York City. Many visitors—enchanted by the town's peace and quiet, fresh spring water from the Blue Mountains, and wholesome food—chose to spend their summer vacations in New Italy. Some, including Italian shoemakers, blacksmiths, barbers, and tailors, deserted New York and Philadelphia to open their shops in Roseto or nearby communities (42).

The new citizens found it an increasing deprivation to be without a church of their own. The nearest Roman Catholic church was in Easton, Pennsylvania, where most Rosetans went for Sunday services, baptisms, weddings, and funerals. The town leaders petitioned Archbishop Ryan, the Roman Catholic bishop of Philadelphia, to establish a mission church in New Italy. His refusal encouraged some Rosetans to embrace the Protestant faith. In 1887, Michelangelo D'Uva, one of the group who had come to America with Dr. Cardo, had moved to New York City and been converted to Protestantism. Visiting New Italy with another Italian convert, Giovanni Gozzolino, a traveling book salesman, D'Uva went from house to house distributing free copies of the Bible and religious pamphlets in the Italian language. He further took advantage of the religious vacuum to persuade many of his compatriots to attend a nearby Presbyterian church at Five Points where there happened to be an Italian pastor, the Reverend A. Arrhigi.

Mr. Arrhigi took a great interest in the immigrants and helped them in many ways, finally managing to persuade the presbytery to open an Evangelical mission in New Italy. The Italians were able to recruit as their first pastor a Lombard Waldensian priest, Emmanuel Tealdo. The first services were held in a shanty with boards laid across for pews and an empty beer keg as a pulpit. There were special services in English on Tuesday afternoons to help the congregation with the language. In addition evening services featured talks by missionaries working in other Italian settlements in the United States. In 1893, with D'Uva's financial assistance, the members constructed a one-room building on a plot of land donated by one of the converts. Thus the Presbyterian mission was chartered with sixty-four members. The same year, and a few days before the Protestant church was completed, a small Catholic church, Our Lady of Mount Carmel, was built. Its establishment stemmed the tide of conversions to Protestantism, but since no priest was available to provide full-time service, the church remained closed for the most part for three years.

Very close to Roseto, in West Bangor, was a second, separately established, predominantly Italian settlement that also lacked a facility for Roman Catholic worship services, although it had a chapel dedicated to Saint Rocco in the home of a lay reader. There was, however, an Italian Episcopal priest, who presided over two mission churches. Many of the West Bangor Italians, viewing the Episcopal liturgy as only slightly different from the Roman Catholic, joined the church and continued as Protestants even after a Catholic church was finally provided (42).

By 1896, Archbishop Ryan had reversed his decision to deny the residents of New Italy their missionary church. He managed to recruit an Italian priest, Father Pasquale de Nisco, from a parish in London, England, to establish a full-time mission in New Italy. Father de Nisco, a cultured and sophisticated man, was able to help the *paesani* with legal, civic, political, and family matters. He exhorted the Italian Presbyterians to return to their mother church or face excommunication, thereby setting off a controversy between the priests and ministers of the area churches that lasted until 1912.

Nine Presbyterian ministers served over the twenty-year period from 1892 to 1912. Then, in the absence of an ordained minister, the pulpit was filled for the next seven years by divinity students (36). By this time the original converts had grown old, some had returned to the Catholic church. During the period of controversy several discontented Presbyterians withdrew to organize the Association of the Bible Students, later known as the Russellites, or Jehovah's Witnesses. There were other trials and tribulations. A libel suit was initiated by one of the priests against the Presbyterian minister in New Italy. Another court case concerned the ownership of a strip of land adjacent to the Presbyterian cemetery.

Father de Nisco inaugurated a comprehensive plan for public improvement that was to serve as a pattern for subsequent progress. He encouraged his parishioners to secure American citizenship, urged parents to send their children to school, established clubs to promote interest in sports, initiated a circulating library, and formed organizations to meet the spiritual needs of specific age groups. The Mutual Aid Society Addolorata looked after the spiritual welfare of adults; the San Luigi Society worked among boys; the Sacred Heart Sodality was directed to mothers and wives; and the Figlie di Maria promoted Christian life among girls.

Father de Nisco began a campaign in the pulpit, in

homes, and in the county court against "Sicilianism." His efforts were effective in reducing petty lawlessness. Most lawbreakers either reformed or left the area. Father de Nisco bought twenty-eight lots around the Catholic church with the idea of constructing a plaza, a parochial school, a hospital, and a cemetery. He encouraged Rosetans to beautify their town after the fashion of the village in Italy. He gave them seeds and bulbs and offered cash prizes for the best flowers. Women cleared the lots with axes and picks, spaded the rocky soil, and planted onions, beans, potatoes, and melons—enough to supply food for the summer and winter months. Fruit trees and grape arbors followed, and within a few years the ample backyards of Roseto's otherwise plain and almost austere homes bloomed with flowering shrubs, fruit trees, and berry bushes and vegetable gardens among patches of lawn.

The priest emphasized the need for cleanliness, often supervising the removal of trash and urging residents to improve their housing. Land values doubled nearly every two years, and the average capital required to begin construction on a house soon rose to four hundred dollars. On Father de Nisco's recommendation the Bangor banks agreed to lend money for building, allowing ten years for repayment. Father de Nisco attempted to improve the lot of the men in the quarries, who were earning only about eight cents an hour, were paid only every three months, and were compelled to trade at company stores. After failing in negotiations with the quarry owners, he organized a labor union, appointing himself as president. When shortly thereafter he called a strike, quarry owners imported one hundred southern blacks as strikebreakers. When the blacks saw the dangerous quarry pits, however, they refused to work and soon returned home. The priest was ultimately successful in increasing workers' wages to $1.50 for a nine-hour day. On another occasion, when a smallpox epidemic erupted in the town, he closed the quarries again by imposing a quarantine on the citizens. In addition, he urged them to become immunized.

Father de Nisco also recommended that the town obtain a wholesale liquor license, for he thought it better that his people should have the light wines and beer to which they were accustomed with their families, "under their own vine and fig trees," rather than frequent the bars in Bangor (2, 13).

Other evidence of civic progress was apparent during Father de Nisco's tenure. It had originally been necessary to travel to Bangor for postal service, for there was no rural postal delivery system. A petition submitted to the Post Office Department for a local branch was granted in 1898. In it the name New Italy was officially replaced with the more euphonious and historically appropriate designation Roseto, Pennsylvania. Another petition to the Northampton County Court requested a special election to divide the electoral seat of Washington Township so that it would no longer be necessary for Rosetans to travel three miles to vote. After that petition was granted as well, the Rosetans began taking an interest in local and national politics. They even ran for local government posts, and some were elected. In 1920, although most Rosetans were Republicans, the Roseto Democratic Club was organized.

A weekly newspaper, *La Stella di Roseto*, established in 1902 in nearby Pen Argyl, provided communication among Italians in Northampton County. It continued publication until its owner's death in 1936. Relationships between Roseto Italians and those living in surrounding towns were further enhanced by the organization in Roseto of the Guglielmo Marconi Pleasure Club in 1903, later known as the Marconi Social Club. The following year, to secure legalization of the club, the members required that the club's officers must be American citizens. A petition for incorporation was granted the club in 1905, after which the building was enlarged and modernized and became a focal point for social activities in the community (2).

Father de Nisco urged the young girls of the community to become wage earners, encouraging many of them to work in the shirt factory in Bangor. Ultimately preferring to keep all the interests of his people concentrated in their town and in their church, however, the priest appealed to the wealthier residents of Roseto to establish their own shirt factory. Finally in 1905 the first such factory was built.

Soon it was producing seventy dozen shirts a day. Shares in the company sold initially at ten dollars each. The girls operating the machines were paid by piecework. Thereby they could supplement their family's incomes by about six to eight dollars a week. While the factory was usually shorthanded because the girls one after another would marry and quit work, it was a standby for hard times and boredom.

By 1905, with a population of nearly two thousand, and with ninety-six registered voters, Roseto potentially controlled the balance of political power in Washington Township. Nevertheless, its schools had the poorest teachers in the township, and its unpaved and unlighted streets were often impassable. Father de Nisco mobilized the voters and soon obtained a new road. By 1906, Roseto, having realized the power of its votes, prepared to incorporate, although some of the citizens, especially the landowners, feared that incorporation would result in higher taxes. Even Father de Nisco was skeptical that his *paesani* could govern themselves. The first petition for incorporation was rejected by the court.

In the midst of Roseto's growing pains the Archbishop of Philadelphia offered Father de Nisco the pastorate of one of that city's well-established churches, where he would find responsibilities less taxing and a respite from his labors. Declining the offer he replied, "I want to die with my boots on."

A second petition for incorporation succeeded, spurred by the vigorous support of younger Rosetans and persuasive editorials in the newspaper, *La Stella di Roseto*. Thereupon, as Roseto became an independent borough, a special election was held in 1912 to select its officials. Roseto thus became the first American municipality governed by Italians. Prior to that time, indeed long before the period of mass immigration, Italian farm colonies had been established. As early as 1844 Italians were market-gardening near Providence, Rhode Island. One of the oldest farm colonies was located in Genoa, Wisconsin, where eight families settled in 1863. Subsequently, several other rural Italian colonies sprang up, including Valdese, North Carolina; Sunnyside and Tontitown, Arkansas; Montebello and Rosati, Missouri; Krebs, Oklahoma; and Bryan, Texas. Father de Nisco, the architect of Roseto, died in 1911 following an appendectomy, and therefore missed by a year the event that gave his town fully independent status. Roseto at the time of his death had grown to 328.5 acres with nearly 300 homes and a total assessed value of $175,000.

In the year following incorporation Columbus Public Grade School was constructed in Roseto, and in 1918 Boy Scout troops were established in the Catholic and Presbyterian churches. The Roseto First National Bank was chartered in 1927, but closed its doors six years later during the Depression. A town hall was dedicated in 1935. De Nisco Park and athletic field were incorporated in 1938. The Salesian Sisters Convent and a parochial kindergarten were built in 1940. The American Legion Martocci-Capobianco

Post No. 750 was organized in 1945. Pius X High School was constructed in 1947. In 1951 the Community Board of Trade (Chamber of Commerce) was formed to better relations between merchants and the Town Council. In 1952 the mayor of Roseto Valfortore in Italy visited the town. In 1953 Our Lady of Mount Carmel Elementary School was completed. In 1962, Roseto celebrated its fiftieth year as an incorporated Italian-American community. The antagonism and scorn of its neighbors had gradually faded over the years. In fact, a degree of admiration and even jealousy of Roseto's prosperity had replaced the old attitudes.

2
Health
and Disease
in Roseto

Widely accepted risk factors for coronary heart disease such as a diet rich in animal fat, cigarette smoking, lack of exercise, diabetes, and hypertension were at least as prevalent in Roseto as in neighboring communities. Nevertheless, we found Rosetans to be favored by a remarkably low death rate from heart attack (myocardial infarction). The incidence of coronary heart disease was clearly lower among Rosetans than among Italian-Americans at large. It was closer, in fact, to that found in rural Italy itself. Despite an equal incidence of the commonly recognized risk factors, the death rate from coronary artery disease in Roseto was less than half that of the surrounding area or of the United States as a whole. In search of an explanation we began in 1961 a series of clinical investigations (5, 7, 9–11, 26, 30, 37, 47, 49, 51, 52).

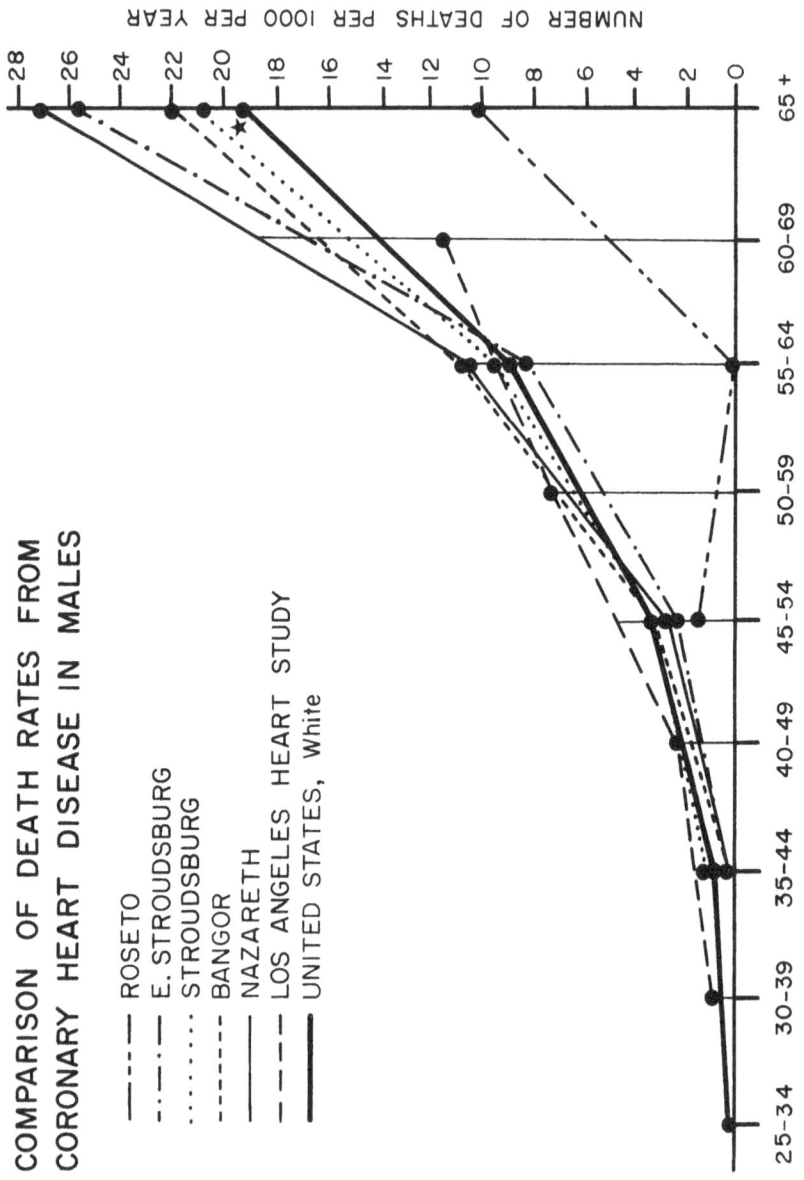

COMPARISON OF DEATH RATES FROM CORONARY HEART DISEASE IN MALES

NUMBER OF DEATHS PER 1000 PER YEAR

- —— ROSETO
- —·—·— E. STROUDSBURG
- ·········· STROUDSBURG
- – – – BANGOR
- NAZARETH
- — — — LOS ANGELES HEART STUDY
- —— UNITED STATES, White

25-34 30-39 35-44 40-49 45-54 50-59 55-64 60-69 65+

★ 65-74

In initial studies we compared mortality statistics among inhabitants of Roseto with those of the four neighboring communities, Nazareth, Bangor, Stroudsburg, and East Stroudsburg, over the seven-year period 1955–61. All death certificates containing cardiac and cardiopulmonary diagnoses, as well as all sudden deaths were collected. The information was verified and supplemented by a review of hospital records with particular attention to electrocardiographic tracings, histories, and autopsy findings. When possible, further strengthening of the data was achieved by checking out patients' records in the offices of their physicians. We found that the death rate from myocardial infarction in Roseto was less than half that of each of the four neighboring towns, where death rates approximated the national figures. The remarkably low death rate from myocardial infarction in the Italian community was most striking among the younger men: during the original seven-year period of study there were no coronary deaths below age forty-seven, while deaths in each decade of life in the surrounding communities matched closely the average figures for the United States. In December, 1961, with a group of physicians, technicians, and dietitians from the University of Oklahoma, we undertook a preliminary medical survey of Roseto. During ten days of daily clinics, approximately 15 per cent of the population over age twenty-five was carefully examined. In addition, electrocardiograms and tests of serum cholesterol, lipoproteins, uric acid, and blood sugar were made on each of the subjects, and from each a thorough dietary history was obtained.

Thereafter, similar detailed observations, plus sociological interviews and questionnaires, were continued in Roseto and in two of the four neighboring towns originally surveyed. One town, Bangor (so named by Welsh immigrants), is immediately adjacent to Roseto, with coextensive streets and a common water supply. Bangor, moreover, is served by the same physicians and the same hospitals as Roseto. Predominantly German Nazareth, the other town studied for comparison, is twelve miles away and is served by a different medical community.

During five successive summers (1962–66), with the cooperation of the mayors and town councils, clinics were set up in the Roseto, Bangor, and Nazareth high schools. Histories, physical examinations, blood chemistries, urine analyses, blood pressures, and electrocardiograms were recorded for 53 percent of the population of Roseto over twenty-five years of age. Included were 269 of 472 men and 271 of 544 women. In Bangor 30 per cent of the population over twenty-five years of age was examined, comprising 487 of 1,715 men and 640 of 2,011 women. In Nazareth 37 percent of the population over twenty-five years of age was examined, comprising 660 of 1,837 men and 789 of 2,050 women.

Table 1 compares the clinic samples in Roseto, Bangor, and Nazareth by age and sex with the age and sex distribution of the three communities and shows

TABLE 1

Representativeness of Clinic Samples in Roseto, Bangor, and Nazareth with Respect to Age and Sex

Age Group	Roseto				Bangor				Nazareth			
	1960 Population	% of Population	Total Clinic Sample	% of Sample	1960 Population	% of Population	Total Clinic Sample	% of Sample	1960 Population	% of Population	Total Clinic Sample	% of Sample
Males												
25–34	109	23	63	23	293	17	91	18	400	22	123	19
35–44	121	26	60	22	380	22	96	20	406	22	142	21
45–54	102	22	63	23	430	25	139	29	410	22	161	24
55–64	69	15	43	16	307	18	85	17	307	17	130	20
65 and over	71	15	40	15	305	18	76	15	314	17	104	16
Total	472		269	57	1,715		487	28	1,837		660	36
Females												
25–34	118	22	55	20	323	16	87	14	405	20	143	18
35–44	143	26	66	24	477	24	144	23	454	22	178	23
45–54	145	27	80	29	458	23	170	26	440	21	175	22
55–64	63	12	48	18	348	17	117	18	365	18	169	21
65 and over	75	14	22	8	405	20	122	19	386	19	124	16
Total	544		271	50	2,011		640	32	2,050		789	38

NOTE: Only individuals age 25 and over were examined in the clinics.

that the samples examined are representative of the population in these respects.

Control for Selection Bias

In order to minimize possible bias in data obtained on a volunteer population, we gathered as controls a random sample of those over twenty-one in Roseto and Nazareth who had not participated in the study. The controls, 36 of 71 from the Roseto list and 201 of 364 from the Nazareth list, agreed to submit to examination. No significant differences between volunteer and random sample populations were found regarding the prevalence of evidence of the diseases studied, except that no persons with myocardial infarction were found in the random sample of men from Roseto or Nazareth. It is surmised that this absence in the randomly selected populations is due to self-segregation into the volunteer population of those who had coronary artery disease, since it was known by the populations of the three communities that this represented a major interest of the investigating team.

Genetic and Ethnic Control

In order to obtain data on people of the same stock who were not inhabitants of Roseto, we accumulated a sample of 350 Italians from other nearby communities and scattered areas of New York, New Jersey, and Pennsylvania who were relatives of Roseto natives or had been born in Roseto and had moved away. Each year, on the last weekend of July, many such relatives and former Rosetans gather in Roseto for the celebration of the Feast of Our Lady of Mount Carmel, the town's patron saint. We were able to enlist their cooperation to undergo the same tests and examinations that were performed on the Rosetans and their neighbors.

Whereas careful study had failed to reveal stigmata of coronary heart disease among Rosetans under age fifty-five, such evidence was common among the representatives of the other populations. We found that the prevalence of evidence of coronary heart disease and the death rate from myocardial infarction among former Rosetans and their families who were living elsewhere in the mid-Atlantic coastal area were relatively high and comparable to the rates among non-Italian Americans. In fact, several deaths from myocardial infarction below age forty-five were documented among those Italians who had been born in Roseto but had lived most of their lives in other communities. Fat intake, exercise habits, cigarette smoking, and serum cholesterol concentration did not appear to be implicated in the discrepancy in the incidence of fatal myocardial infarction between Rosetans and their relatives living elsewhere. Neither could the relatively low incidence of death from myocardial infarction in Roseto be explained by ethnic or genetic factors.

Among possible social explanations one might infer

that the striking increase in stigmata of coronary artery disease among Rosetans who had moved away to live elsewhere may relate to a dissatisfaction with opportunities on the local scene. The desire for change and self-improvement may suggest that coronary disease could be accelerated and intensified among those who are upwardly mobile with respect to education and type of job and who, in addition, are geographically mobile. Indeed, Frederick H. Epstein observed from a comprehensive review of studies of coronary heart disease throughout the world that, "in general, the frequency of coronary heart disease is greater among groups with higher socio-economic standards" (15). He also noted that the urbanization of rural areas was often accompanied by a rise in mortality of arteriosclerotic heart disease and that occupational and geographic mobility appear to be associated with a high incidence of coronary disease.

Apart from the Epstein study and a few others, epidemiological surveys of coronary heart disease have attributed geographic differences in mortality and morbidity to differing dietary practices characteristic of the locality, although physical exercise and cigarette smoking have been accorded some attention. While a few investigators have explored the effects of psychological stresses, the possible relevance of social and cultural patterns has been largely neglected. Since most reports on localities with very low rates of coronary heart disease lack any information concerning the prevailing culture and way of life, we undertook to explore that dimension by marshaling what is known of the social structures and customs of the countries from which published reports have come (10). From this we learned that the social patterns of areas of the world with a low prevalence of coronary heart disease are characterized by stability and predictability. In general we found that in those communities each person has a clearly defined role in the social scheme, man-woman relationships are firmly established, and the elderly have an important place. Indeed, low prevalence and incidence of coronary heart disease correlates better with these features in a society than with the absence or low incidence of any of the conventionally accepted risk factors. Thus our findings in Roseto appear to gain a measure of confirmation from studies of other communities scattered over the world.

Conventionally Recognized Risk Factors

The original data on eating habits mentioned above were extended in Roseto in order to verify, insofar as possible, the dietary patterns. A team of dietitians spent two weeks in Roseto observing the buying patterns in local grocery stores, talking with the grocers about the food stocked and sold, eating many meals in the homes of Rosetans, obtaining weekly diaries from several representative families, and finally analyzing actual food samples collected from several families at mealtimes (21). Confirming the data from dietary histories, this on-site investigation revealed that Rosetans consumed at least as much animal fat as their neighbors or the average American did.

Among Rosetans the age-adjusted prevalence of diabetes was found to be 26 per 1,000 men and 37 per 1,000 women. For Nazareth the figures were 44 and 30 per 1,000 men and women, respectively. Bangor had the highest prevalence of diabetes, 94 per 1,000 men and 102 per 1,000 women.

Obesity was clearly more prevalent among Rosetans than among the inhabitants of the other towns or even among the Italians from elsewhere. Obesity in Rosetan men was most prevalent among the young and declined with age, while among the women the age trend was reversed.

At the time of the examination an elevated blood-pressure reading of 150/90 or above was encountered more frequently among Rosetan men of all ages than among men in the other two towns or among Italian men from other parts of the eastern United States. A single blood-pressure reading is not significant for a diagnosis of hypertension, however, and the Roseto men did not differ from those in the other communities with respect to other physical or laboratory abnormalities related to hypertension. Blood pressure did not differ strikingly among the various groups of women.

Other Diseases

Evidence of peptic ulcer was sought from 86 percent of Rosetans age twenty-one and over. Of 898 respondents 61, or 6.7 percent, reported a positive history of peptic ulcer. Their physicians were able to confirm the diagnosis in 33, roughly half of them. Table 2

TABLE 2

Age-Specific Rates of Peptic Ulcer in Roseto

Age Groups	Rate	Number of Cases	Number in Sample	Number of Expected Cases
		Males		
25–34	.0138	2	109	4.15
35–44	.0413	5	121	10.90
45–54	.0490	5	102	12.10
55–64	.0870	6	69	11.48
65 and over	.0914	4	71	13.34
Total		22	472	51.98
	Standardized rate = 5.116 per 100			
		Females		
25–34	. . .	0	118	0
35–44	.0140	2	143	3.69
45–54	.0345	5	145	8.52
55–64	.0635	4	63	8.38
65 and over	. . .	0	75	0
Total		11	544	20.59
	Standardized rate = 2.027 per 100			

NOTE: The total population of Roseto over 25 years of age was used as a standard. The ages of males and females were comparable. The female rate is 39.6 per cent of the male rate.

shows the age-specific rates of peptic ulcer in Roseto for males and females. It is noted that the standardized rate for females (2.027 per 100) is less than the expected number of cases in the standard population and is 39.6 percent of the male rate. Although comparative data for Bangor and Nazareth were not obtained, this observation may significantly reflect personality characteristics among Rosetans. Fewer of them may be striving, driving people who feel unsupported in their efforts to get ahead than one might encounter in the average American community.

The records of each of the public and private psychiatric institutions and of seven psychiatrists in private practice in Northampton County were examined to ascertain the number of persons from the communities of Roseto, Bangor, and Nazareth who received psychiatric treatment for the first time during the period 1950 to 1960 (6).

The state institution for the mentally ill in Northampton County in which residents of Roseto, Bangor, and Nazareth were hospitalized is situated in Allentown, Pennsylvania. There are three general categories of admissions to this hospital, as provided for in the Pennsylvania Mental Health Act of 1951: voluntary, involuntary, and court commitment. Most admissions to this hospital are involuntary and are primarily psychotic patients admitted for indeterminate detention. Admission requires the support of certificates from two physicians and usually a statement from a relative. All patients admitted for the first time to this

TABLE 3

Average Annual Rates per 100,000 Population of Publicly and Privately Treated Mental Illness in Nazareth, Bangor, and Roseto by Age and Sex, 1950–60

| | Nazareth (pop = 6,019) | | | | | | Bangor (pop = 5,908) | | | | | | Roseto (pop = 1,653) | | | | | |
| | Male | | | Female | | | Male | | | Female | | | Male | | | Female | | |
Age Groups	N =	Rate	S.E.	N =	Rate	S.E.	N =	Rate	S.E.	N =	Rate	S.E.	N =	Rate	S.E.	N =	Rate	S.E.
Under 15	16	192.9	48.2	7	90.5	34.2		52.1	26.0	6	84.3	34.4	0	0.0		1	44.3	44.3
15–24	15	365.6	94.2	33	723.0	125.4		381.1	101.6	19	463.1	106.0	2	176.5	124.7	1	79.1	79.0
25–34	33	723.0	125.4	41	835.7	130.0		342.1	91.3	28	599.0	112.8	4	273.4	136.5	7	441.9	166.7
35–44	24	525.7	107.0	37	747.5	122.4		296.7	79.2	26	474.6	92.9	0	0.0		4	236.1	117.9
45–54	22	536.2	114.0	22	496.3	105.5		447.8	99.9	18	387.8	91.2	3	296.4	170.9	8	649.4	228.8
55–64	25	806.0	160.5	20	539.5	120.3		577.7	132.1	15	391.8	101.0	2	324.7	229.2	1	142.0	141.9
65 and over	32	996.3	175.2	28	709.0	133.5		283.1	94.2	14	347.7	92.8	3	395.3	227.8	2	275.5	194.5
Crude rates		522.8			549.0			302.3			372.0			161.1			253.7	
Age-adjusted rates		505.8			518.0			289.0			351.2			162.2			234.6	

NOTE: Rates were computed using the mean of the 1950 and 1960 U.S. Census. The ages of males and females are comparable. The Pennsylvania male population was used as a standard.

hospital during the period 1950 to 1960 who resided in Roseto, Bangor, or Nazareth at the time of admission were included in the study. The place of residence, sex, age, marital status, diagnosis, length of hospitalization, date of initial contact with the institution, and previous psychiatric treatment were recorded in each case. The records of the Neuropsychiatric Unit of Allentown General Hospital were also examined for first admissions from the three communities from 1950 to 1960. Eleven psychiatrists engaged in full-time private practice were consulted. Two of the psychiatrists had begun their practice after 1960 and therefore had no data relevant to the study. Two other psychiatrists were unwilling to participate. The remaining seven psychiatrists provided the age, sex, date of initial contact, and diagnosis of all patients seen by them from the three communities during the specified period of time.

Table 3 shows the average annual rates of public and privately treated mental illness in Nazareth, Bangor, and Roseto for the years 1950 to 1960. While there were differences from decade to decade for the three towns, the over-all rate for treated mental illness in Bangor was nearly twice that in Roseto, and in Nazareth almost three times that in Roseto. The age-adjusted rate for admission to Allentown State Hospital that for Rosetans by a factor of nearly two. There were no male first admissions from Roseto under age sixty-five.

Table 4 shows the diagnoses of first admissions to

TABLE 4

Percentage and Number of First Admissions to Allentown State Hospital from Nazareth, Bangor, and Roseto by Diagnosis Compared with First Admissions to all Other Pennsylvania State Hospitals, 1950–60

| | Allentown State Hospital | | | | | | All Other Pennsylvania State Hospitals | |
| | Nazareth | | Bangor | | Roseto | | | |
Diagnosis	%	N =	%	N =	%	N =	%	N =
Chronic brain syndrome with senile brain disease or circulatory disorders	46	31	28	13	57	4	30	18,836
Chronic brain syndrome with central nervous system syphilis	0	0	7	3	0	0	2	1,130
Chronic brain syndrome with alcoholism or drugs	3	2	4	2	0	0	2	1,344
Chronic brain syndrome, other*	2	1	4	2	0	0	4	2,613
Manic depressive psychoses	4	3	9	4	0	0	3	2,115
Schizophrenic reactions	27	18	31	14	29	2	30	18,524
Involutional psychotic reactions	3	2	4	2	14	1	4	2,417
Psychoneuroses and character disorders	3	2	9	4	0	0	14	8,728
Mental deficiencies	10	7	2	1	0	0	4	2,232
Other	2	1	2	1	0	0	7	4,176
Total		67		46		7		62,115

*Including chronic brain syndrome with no specific type indicated.

35

TABLE 5

Diagnoses of Private Psychiatric Patients from Nazareth, Bangor, and Roseto, 1950–60

	Nazareth		Bangor		Roseto	
Diagnosis	%	N =	%	N =	%	N =
Chronic brain syndrome with senile brain disease or circulatory disorders	4	13	3	6	3	1
Chronic brain syndrome with central nervous system syphilis	3	1	1	2	0	(
Chronic brain syndrome with alcoholism or drugs	1	2	0	0	0	(
Chronic brain syndrome, other*	11	34	5	9	3	1
Manic depressive psychoses	2	7	5	1	3	1
Schizophrenic reactions	9	27	14	25	13	4
Involutional psychotic reactions	12	37	12	21	9	:
Psychoneuroses and character disorders	48	147	55	100	56	18
Mental deficiencies	1	2	3	5	0	(
Unclassified and other	11	34	7	12	13	4
Total		304		181		32

*Including chronic brain syndrome with no specific type indicated.

36

Allentown State Hospital from Nazareth, Bangor, and Roseto in comparison with those of all other Pennsylvania state hospitals. First admissions from Bangor and Nazareth did not differ greatly by diagnosis, nor did they differ to any great extent by diagnosis from the first admissions to other Pennsylvania state hospitals. However, all the Roseto patients fell into three of the diagnostic categories: senility, schizophrenia, and involutional psychosis.

Table 5 records the diagnoses of private psychiatric patients from the three towns from 1950 to 1960. As would be expected, over half of the private patients from all three towns were diagnosed as having psychoneurotic and character disorders. No cases of mental deficiency appear among public or private patients from Roseto, owing in part to the custom of keeping the mentally deficient at home and to the existence of a country day school in Bangor for mentally retarded children. Of the 100 children attending this school, 24 percent were from Bangor and 11 percent were from Roseto.

Although the information on coronary heart disease was periodically updated, no further checks on peptic ulcer and mental disease are at present available. Nevertheless, the relatively low prevalence of peptic ulcer, senile dementia, and certain other mental illnesses may be linked, like the low rate of coronary heart disease, to the social structure, the Rosetan way of life.

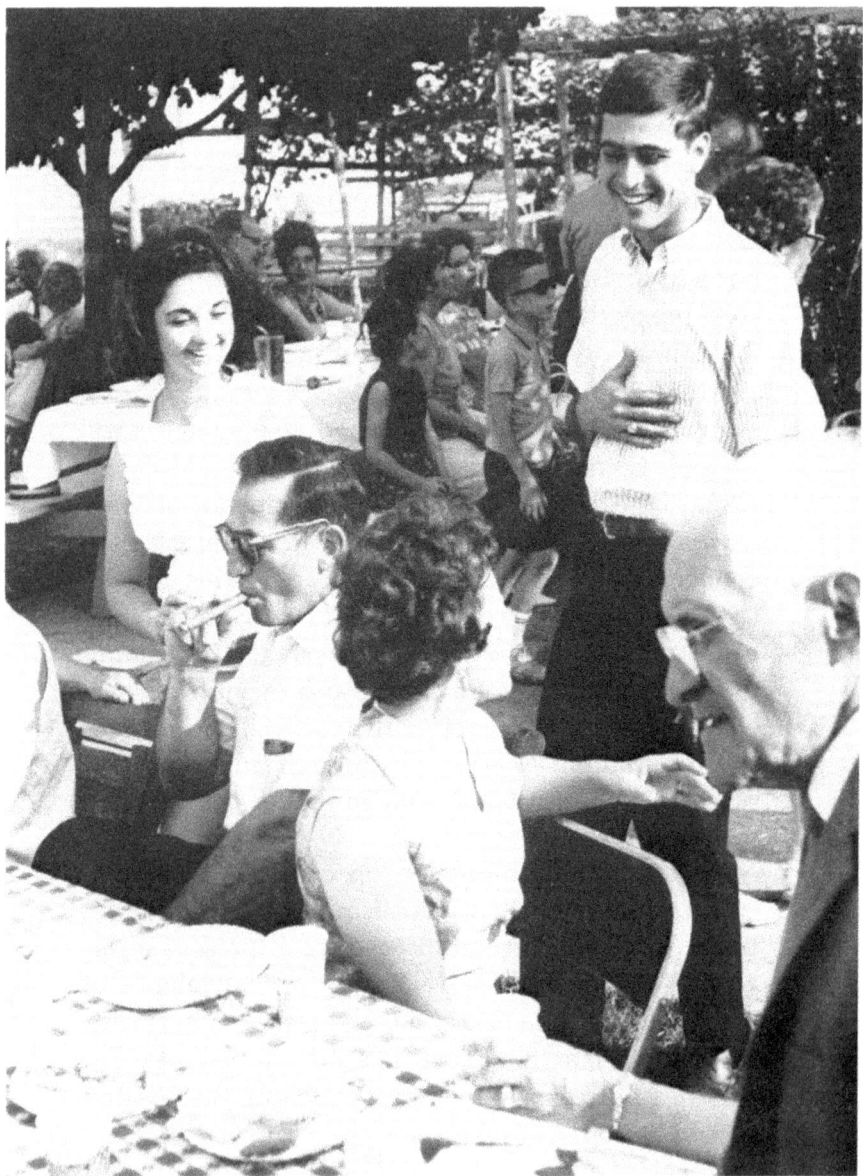

A backyard celebration of a high-school graduation in Roseto.

3
The Rosetan
Way
of Life

As already emphasized in Chapter 1, the Italian immigrant founders of Roseto were not accepted socially by their Anglo-Saxon neighbors. Nor did they have equal opportunity in respect to skilled or semiskilled jobs in the quarries where they obtained employment. The English and the Welsh considered the skilled jobs their peculiar prerogative because they or their ancestors, having learned the trade in the British Isles, were "qualified." The Italians were only good enough to "work in the hole or throw out the rubbish." They were paid eight cents an hour for a ten-hour day. Paydays came every three months, and in the interims they were required to shop at company stores (42). They were thus forced to establish their own enclave and to look out for their own welfare. As

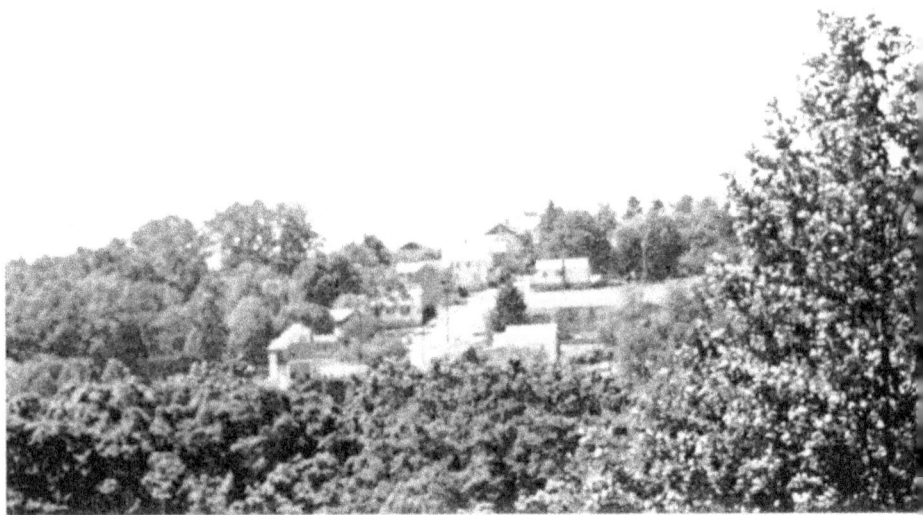

Roseto, Pennsylvania, 1965.

they met the challenge with pride and determination, the result was an accentuation of the natural tendency of southern Italians to maintain close family and community ties. Valletta reports that within two generations they developed a parochial grammar and high school, built up the garment industry to a dominant position in the area, and established Catholic and Presbyterian churches, as well as many clubs and organizations dedicated to mutual help (42). Ultimately Roseto emerged as a buoyant, fun-loving community that was more enterprising, more self-

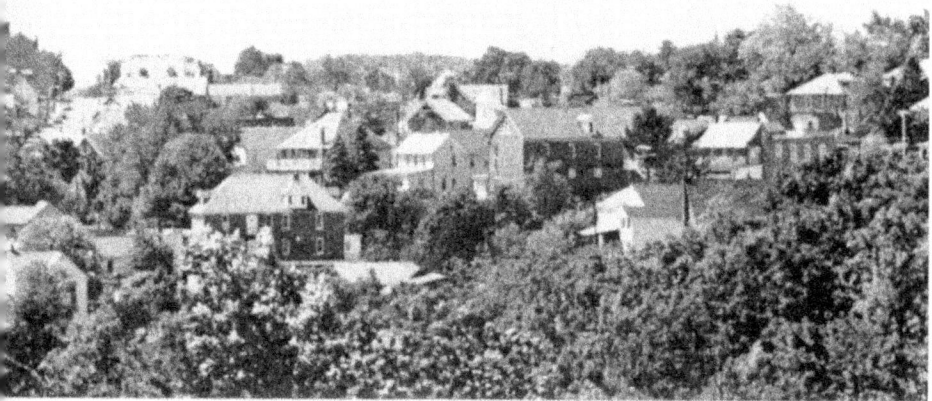

sufficient, more optimistic, and more prosperous than its neighbors. The persistent cohesive and mutually supportive quality of the town was evident from such frequent comments of Rosetans as:

People in other places live too fast. It's nice and quiet around here. People around here are friendly.

I like the people all sociable and with a good heart, religious, like a big family all raised together.

Where else can you go where your friends and relatives all help out in time of trouble? Everyone trusts everyone else.

Our first sociological study of Roseto revealed that crises and problems were coped with jointly by family members with support from relatives and friends. Following a death in the family, interfamilial differences were forgotten, and the bereaved received food and money from relatives and friends, who at times temporarily assumed responsibility for the care of the children of the bereaved. When financial problems arose, relatives and friends rallied to the aid of the family, and in instances of abrupt, extreme financial loss the community itself assumed responsibility for helping the family. Personal and family problems were usually worked out with the help of other clan members and often the priest. The elderly were cared for in the homes of their kin and were usually institutionalized only when extreme physical and mental deterioration prohibited further home care. In cases of illegitimacy, divorce, or mental retardation the affected person was normally cared for at home.

Even today the major responsibility for family problems in Roseto falls upon, or is assumed by, the unmarried females or other family members with no children. Several single women in the community have assumed the role of pillar of the family in lieu of marriage and have undertaken the primary responsibility for caring for their elderly parents. Usually such a woman is the "strongest" member of the family. Common attitudes among these "pillars" are the maintenance of close family ties, the security derived from their religion, and the knowledge that the respected people in the community are on their side. These attitudes are considered essential in coping with family crises. "When you have these things," one woman said, "then you can carry your cross."

Location

Roseto, seventy-five miles north of Philadelphia and about seventy-five miles west of New York City, is situated in Northampton County, in the slate belt of east-central Pennsylvania, about fifteen miles north of Easton, the county seat. Access roads lead from the north through the Blue Mountains, the Delaware Water Gap and West Bangor; from the east across the Delaware River at Portland, Pennsylvania, and from there through Mount Bethel; and more directly from the south by Highway 611 north from Easton along the winding scenic Delaware River to Martins Creek. At Martins Creek the short journey continues on Highway 712 over narrow winding roads through several small townships into Bangor, Roseto's closest neighbor. In Bangor huge heaps of slate rubble tower over the buildings of the city. The initial impression of Bangor, with its one- and two-story frame houses and small concentrated business district, is one of an old northeastern industrial town. The road to Roseto rises sharply at the northern edge of the Bangor business district along Martins Creek. Viewed from the east, Roseto appears terraced with homes nestled on the slopes. The highest and lowest elevations are, respectively, 720 and 620 feet above sea level.

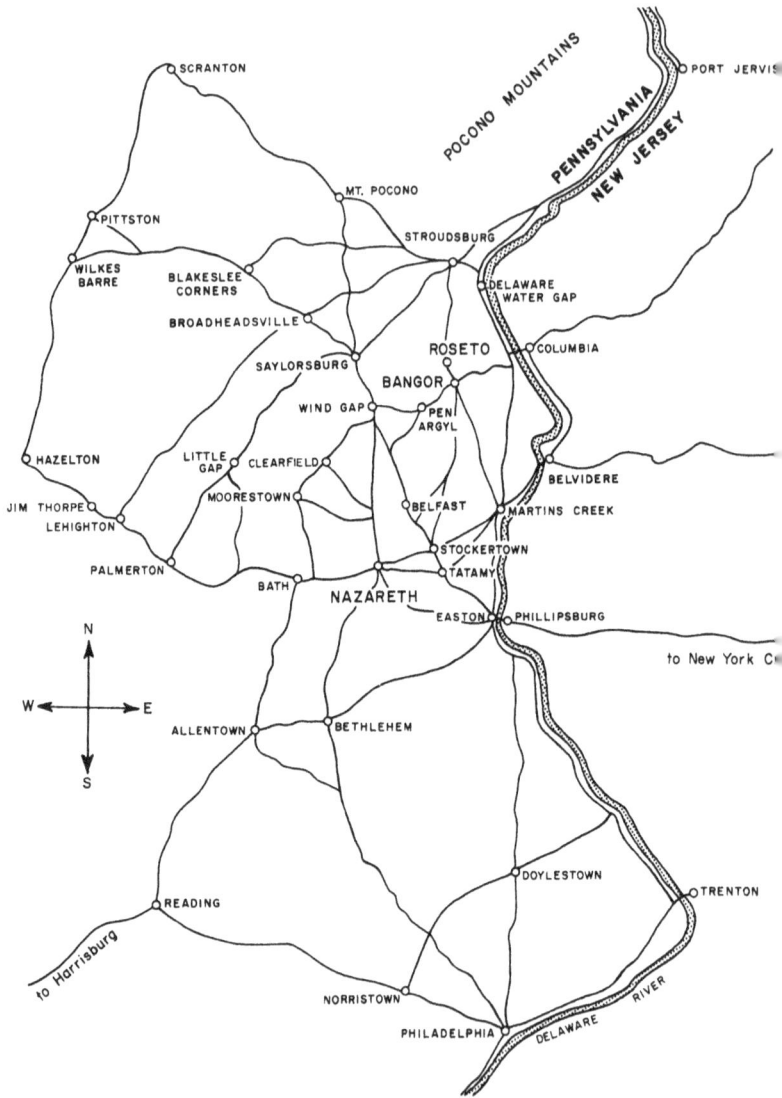

Roseto and its environs.

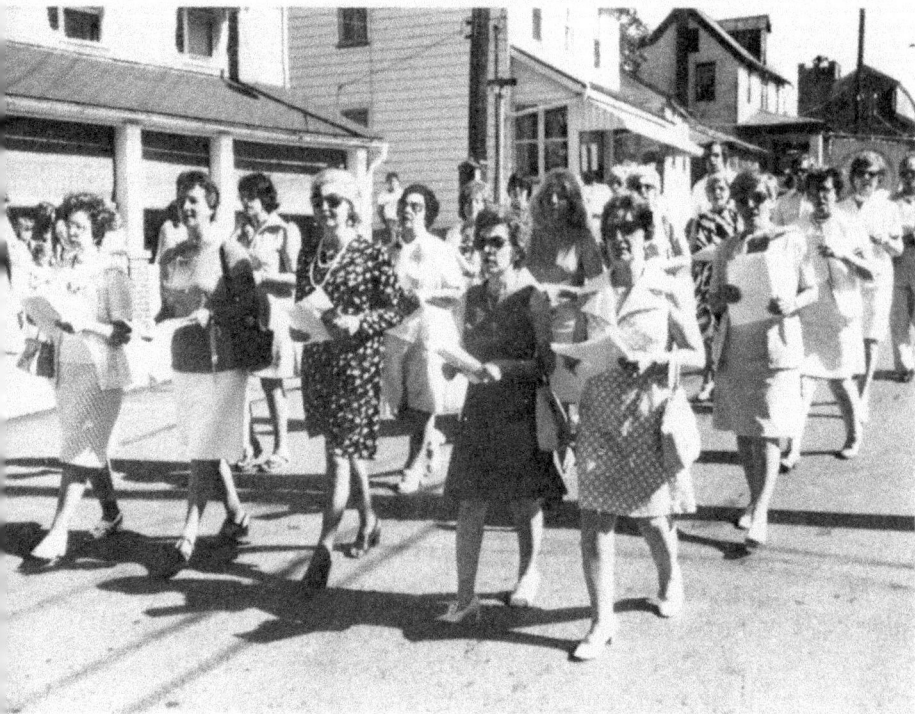

The annual procession honoring Our Lady of Mount Carmel on Garibaldi Avenue. The houses in the background are built close to one another and to the street as was the custom in Roseto till the 1960's.

The town covers a land area of one-half square mile. The narrow cement streets, for the most part bearing Italian names, are patched here and there with asphalt. The main street, Garibaldi Avenue, connects the northern and southern boundaries of the town. Here the houses are close together and near the street, so that residents sitting on their porches can talk readily with neighbors and passersby while they watch the town's activities. The lots are deep and narrow with lawn and garden space behind the houses. Gardens and a few grape arbors are evident, especially at the homes of the older residents.

The assessed valuation of real estate in Roseto in 1970 was about $3.5 million. Of the 350 homes in the town—mainly two-story frame dwellings—some were divided into apartments occupied by various families of one clan. Others, mainly along Garibaldi Avenue and adjacent streets, contained Roseto's thirty small businesses. Italian bakeries operated by a pair of cousins occupied the basements of two of the homes, where large bread loaves, varieties of pizza, fish pie, pasta, and pretzels were baked. The one meat market in Roseto was also on Garibaldi Avenue. The five restaurants in the town and three adjoining bars all occupied the first floors of their owner's residences. Sixteen blouse mills scattered throughout the town constituted the remaining local industry. Altogether, in Roseto and immediately adjacent areas, there were thirty of these mills.

The Characteristics of the People

As described by Clement Valletta, a young social scientist born in Roseto, the community evolved from the well-defined culture of southern Italian peasants, *contadini,* with their firm belief in and fear of super-

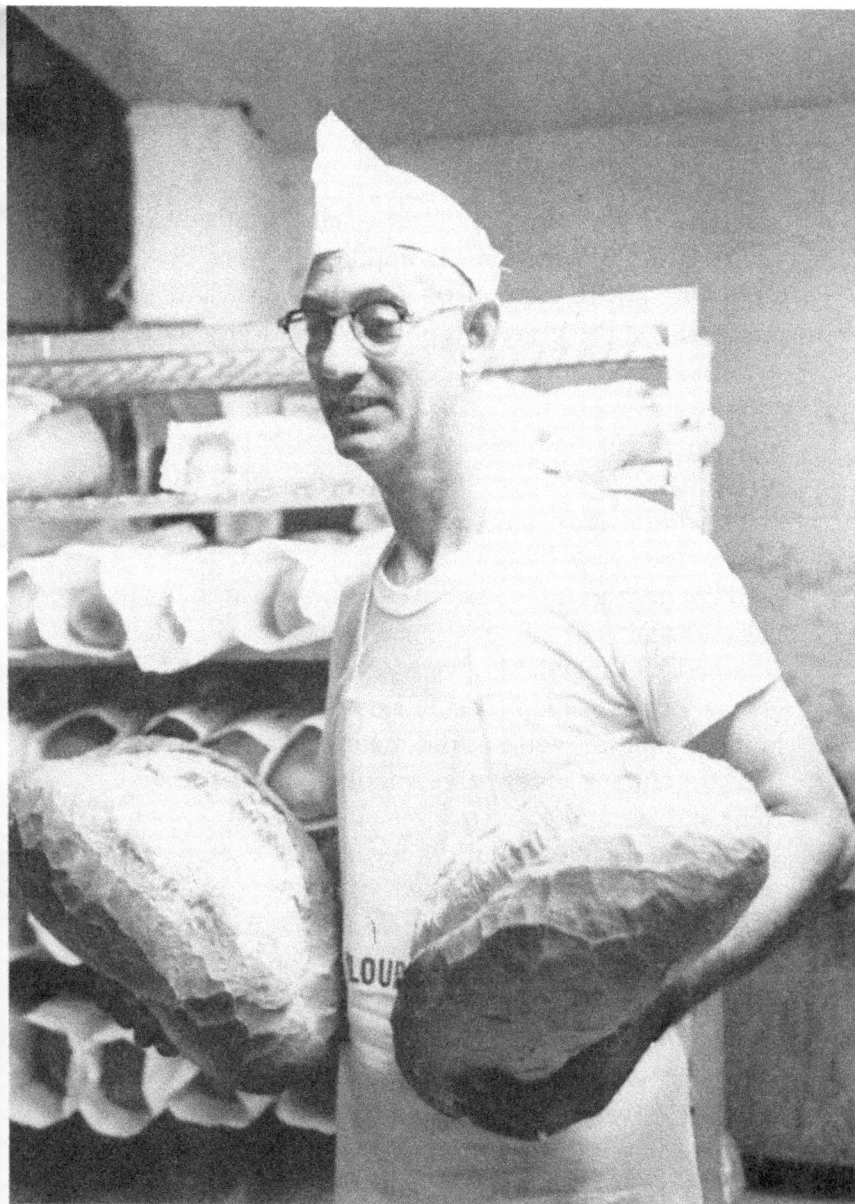

One of Roseto's bakers
(photograph by Steve Schapiro).

natural forces set in motion especially by strong desires, or *voli*. These supernatural beliefs were closely
intertwined with their deep religious faith and dependence on the good will of the Virgin Mary. Unfa-
vorable circumstances associated with *malocchio*, the
evil eye, were brought on by envious, evil, or vindic-
tive *voli* of others. The explanation of such natural
phenomena as storms, floods, and droughts lay not
in a scientific approach but in intense human desires,
God, or fate. According to Valletta: "When times were
hard the immigrant knew it was useless to argue with
fate. With almost a Greek sense of destiny, Rosetans
accepted the inevitable even while they prayed for
Divine intercession." The Rosetans felt as much at
home in their universe as did medieval men who saw
their firmament alive with symbols of good and evil,
right and wrong (42).

At the time of our study a few older Rosetans still
made their own wine, half of which they gave away
to friends and relatives. They made the first batch in
November from imported California Concord grapes.
They often made a second wine from grapes they
grew in the backyards of their own homes. They grew
Italian lettuce, cabbage, green peppers, onions, peas,
beans, endives, radishes, eggplant, tomatoes, corn,
beets, cucumbers, figs, peaches, pears, apples,
pumpkins, cherries, plums, parsley, oregano, mint,
and other spices in their backyard gardens. They
canned much of the produce for the winter.

During the day the community was quiet and had

the appearance of a ghost town because almost all Rosetans of both sexes and all ages had jobs. They gathered in the evening at the social clubs or in their homes. The behavior of teenagers was remarkably restrained. Their gathering place was Mary's Luncheonette. The duties of the local police were confined largely to directing traffic for funerals and the Festival of Our Lady of Mount Carmel. The fire department, with only a rare small blaze to fight, engaged in frequent drills to keep their newly acquired modern fire truck in working order.

TABLE 6

Population of Roseto, 1920–70

Year	Total Population
1920	1,643
1930	1,746
1940	1,778
1950	1,676
1960	1,630
1970	1,538

SOURCE: U.S. Census of Population. No census data are available for 1910 since Roseto was not incorporated as a borough until 1912.

From its first census in 1920 to 1950, Roseto's population remained approximately stable. Since then there has been a decline in population (Table 6) and

TABLE 7

Number of Resident Live Births and Total Deaths for Roseto, Bangor, and Nazareth, 1961–71
(rate per 1,000 estimated mid-year population)

Year	Roseto				Bangor				Nazareth			
	Number of Births	Rate	Number of Deaths	Rate	Number of Births	Rate	Number of Deaths	Rate	Number of Births	Rate	Number of Deaths	Rate
1961	21	12.9	11	6.7	81	14.1	64	11.1	95	15.3	71	11.5
1962	27	16.7	14	8.6	96	16.8	67	11.7	124	20.2	86	14.0
1963	19	11.8	13	8.0	84	14.8	63	11.1	121	19.8	87	14.2
1964	22	13.7	13	8.1	114	20.2	100	17.7	130	21.4	88	14.5
1965	26	16.3	18	11.3	83	14.7	77	13.7	103	17.0	90	14.9
1966	34	21.4	22	13.9	85	15.2	81	14.5	104	17.3	81	13.5
1967	11	6.9	22	13.9	72	12.9	67	12.0	100	16.7	101	16.9
1968	17	10.8	11	7.0	68	12.3	87	15.7	107	18.0	75	12.6
1969	20	12.8	15	9.6	85	15.4	65	11.8	94	15.9	77	13.0
1970	11	7.0	13	8.3	71	13.0	74	13.5	104	17.7	66	11.2
1971	17	11.0	16	10.3	62	11.4	77	14.1	81	13.9	91	15.6

SOURCE: Department of Health, Commonwealth of Pennsylvania, Harrisburg.

TABLE 8

Percentage Distribution of Rosetans by Sex and Age

Age	Males N =	%	Females N =	%	Totals N =	%
21–30	58	14	75	15	133	15
31–44	115	29	143	29	258	29
45–54	114	28	134	27	248	28
55–64	58	14	89	18	147	16
65 and over	58	14	54	11	112	12
Totals	403		495		898	
Mean Age	47.2		46.4			

especially in the birth rate (Table 7). Vital statistics for 1960 include a mean age for males of 47.2 years and a mean age for females of 46.4 years. In contrast to most American communities, life expectancy for men in Roseto is slightly longer than that for women. Indeed, we found a few more widowers than widows in the town, although over all, females outnumbered males five to four (see Table 8 for life expectancies of all age groups 21 years and older).

Further demographic data on the population of Roseto revealed:

74 percent married once

2 percent married more than once

2 percent separated or divorced

8 percent widowed (more men than women)

14 percent single (more women than men)
Mean age at marriage for men 24.6 years
Mean age at marriage for women 22.1 years

Clement Valletta observes that, after nearly one hundred years of exposure to American traditions,

they still cling to their Italian traditions in the hierarchical family structure; they still try to avoid community malediction for their family by admonishing their children with the words, "What will people think"; they still worship through the Madonna and Jesus; and even the few who gamble and the many who follow sports address whatever fate has made them win or lose. The town has become a group of clans (interrelated families), each with a patriarch and matriarch, much like the figureheads of a European nation; a directing prime minister, who is usually a blouse contractor; and a cabinet made up of brothers and sisters, at least one of whom has some advanced education and is in charge of protocol and new ideas. Thus familial forms of the nuclear immigrant family have been extended to the clan made up of the surviving immigrants, their married children, and the grandchildren. Although a study in itself, clans are dominant if there are several brothers having status as contractors or professionists. A male in-law who is not so prestigious may be drawn into his wife's clan. Familial forms have also been extended into the blouse factories, clubs, and organizations (42).

The cornerstone of Rosetan life is the family. Families in turn are tied to each other through inter-marriage to form "clans," one or another of which embraces most Rosetans. Family traditions provide a buffer in times of crisis and a source of stability for the community. They largely dictate individual behavior in relation to community functions and even outside activities. Family celebrations still mark every important event in the development of the children: first communion, graduation from high school, engagement and marriage. Birthdays, anniversaries and special days of all sorts also provide cause for celebration. Family and friends gather in the spacious back lawn of one of the houses for a feast prepared and served by the ladies. Pitchers of red wine poured over peaches are circulated to the company along with a generous supply of sausages, pizzas, and a variety of other Italian delicacies.

Until recently most Rosetan families had six or more children, but now the average is one to three. We found that 12 percent of families were childless. More than 25 per cent of Rosetan couples lived with parents or other family members, and more than half of the single, widowed, or divorced persons lived with family members. Most infants were breast-fed by their mothers but were mothered by many females in the close family unit, including older sisters, aunts, grandmothers, and even cousins. As they grew up, the children played mainly with their own relatives and nearby neighbors.

Most Rosetans are second- or third-generation Italians, although there are now a few fourth-generation inhabitants. Those who have married non-Italians make up approximately 15 per cent of the population; most of them live on the periphery of the town and

TABLE 9

Percentage Distribution of the Population of Roseto on the Family Solidarity Index, 1966

1.	Subject is living with spouse	74
2.	Subject is of the same ethnicity as spouse	74
3.	Subject is of the same religion as spouse	77
4.	Subject has lived in Roseto all of life	55
5.	Spouse has lived in Roseto all of life	42
6.	Children living with parents	69
7.	Subject and spouse spend time with others	19
8.	All children live at home	62
9.	Children are married to Italians	58
10.	Subject turns to family with problems	70
11.	All siblings live in Roseto	17
12.	Subject attends family reunions	34

are often excluded from the mainstream of Rosetan life.

In order to assess the degree of cohesiveness in families, we incorporated a family solidarity index into the survey. While the scores differed from family to family, the over-all score indicated a generally high degree of cohesiveness among families, as shown in Table 9. The table lists the findings on the twelve criteria that make up the family solidarity index and demonstrates the highly cohesive nature of the community of Roseto.

The Young People

Interviews with teenagers in Roseto and Bangor began in 1963. They were asked questions regarding their attitudes toward Roseto, their educational aspirations, and their involvement in school and community activities. Roseto teenagers displayed a higher degree of family solidarity than Bangor Italian teenagers and Bangor non-Italian teenagers. Both Roseto and Bangor Italian teenagers, however, belonged to fewer organized peer groups than did the Bangor non-Italian teenagers. Thus Italian youth in general were primarily "homebound," associating with peers of their own ethnic group rather than joining school or community organizations.

There was very little evidence of adolescent rebellion in Roseto. Teenagers for the most part were tractable and well behaved. Nevertheless, they expressed a certain restlessness, dissatisfaction with opportunities in Roseto, and even the rejection of the prevailing mores. The Roseto teenagers expressed aspirations to live as middle-class Americans but were confronted with the limitations in achieving this by remaining in Roseto. They recognized the need for independence from enclave life to achieve their middle-class aspirations, yet were ambivalent regarding the possible success of their independent efforts and the degree of satisfaction that middle-class rewards would provide as opposed to their present way of life. We learned that many young Rosetans who left their community for college educations and specialized jobs did not return to live in Roseto.

Education appeared to be a major force for changing attitudes among Rosetan teenagers. Rosetan and

Bangor Italian parents encouraged their young people to pursue college and higher education. They took pride in the fact that more than 150 individuals from their ethnic group had entered semiprofessional or professional occupations since the turn of the century.

Most Rosetan teenagers felt that after specialized training they would not fit in the Rosetan culture. To quote one of them:

There is very little excitement. No industry, which is the reason for young college graduates to abandon this town. There is no place to get ahead. Other than the mills, there is nothing a person can do for a living. The children in Roseto have a chance for a good education, but it is hard to live in Roseto if you acquire a specialized education. All Rosetans have a higher goal, but the old people want to keep things the way they are used to.

Yet some Rosetan teenagers seemed ambivalent about compromising their way of life, and some voiced concern for the future of their town, as illustrated in the following quotes from three Rosetan teenagers:

I think Roseto is a fairly good town in which to live. There is a deep security in knowing when problems are to be faced. Most people in town can rely on certain members of the family to help them solve these problems. There are many opportunities for children to develop socially because of the closeness or affinity people have for one another. The town also faces serious problems. Some of these are related to the lack of sufficient job opportunities for men. Because of the lack of well-paying job opportunities, women must work and men must usually leave the town to find better jobs. I think that this problem leaves much to be desired in the cultural development and broad-mindedness of most of the people in the town. Most of the people are well off financially, but they must work too hard for what they have. I think the people are very happy in the town. They have a firm belief in God and desire better conditions for their children.

I think Roseto is a very good place in which to live, but I do not think I will live here after my education is completed. I say this because I do not expect to find a job in this area. However, I feel I have gained much by growing up in Roseto, and I would like to live in a town similar to it in size and location. Knowing many of the people in the town definitely has its faults, but it also has its advantages, which I feel outweigh the former. I am proud of my Italian heritage and the fact that many Rosetans are now very successful, although they had little to start with.

I feel safe and completely happy being in Roseto; for some strange reason I do not want to leave Roseto. It is peaceful. There are no gangs; one is brought up wholesome. The people are sociable. The fact that most of the residents are Italians provides a unified community.

Local Industry and Occupations

Slate mining, initially the principal industry of Roseto and Bangor, began to decline in the 1930's. As the men demanded higher and higher wages to work in the hazardous quarry pits, the market for slate decreased. From 1930 to 1970 the number of active quarries in the area diminished from about fifteen to three. A few Rosetan men still work in those quarries,

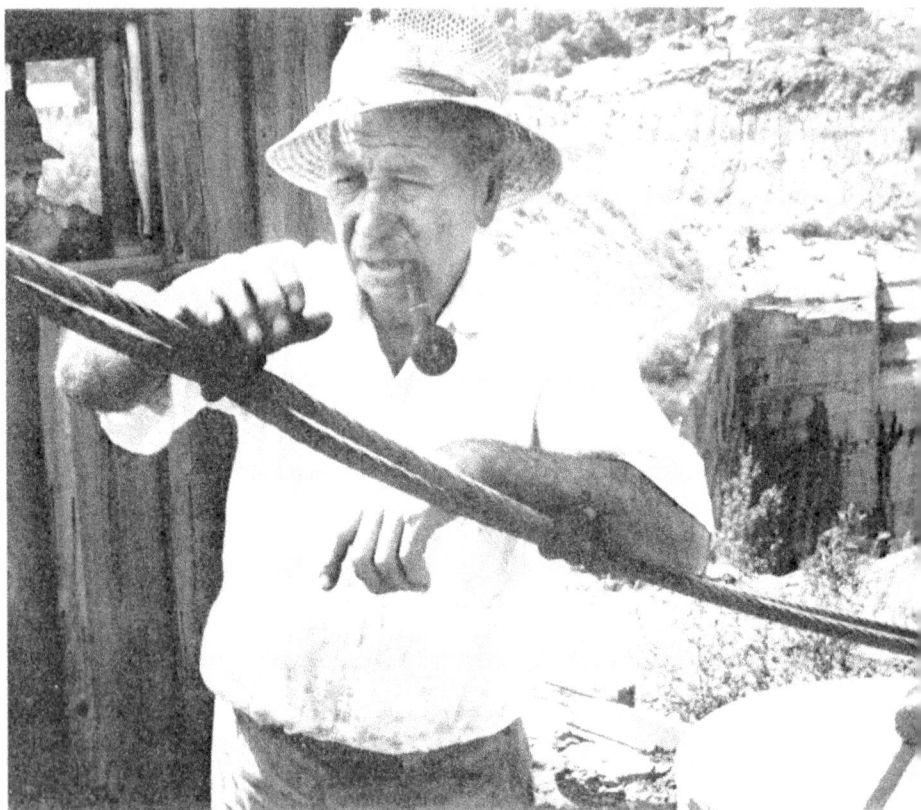

Operating a mechanical hoist in a Bangor slate quarry.

Men being lowered to quarry slate.

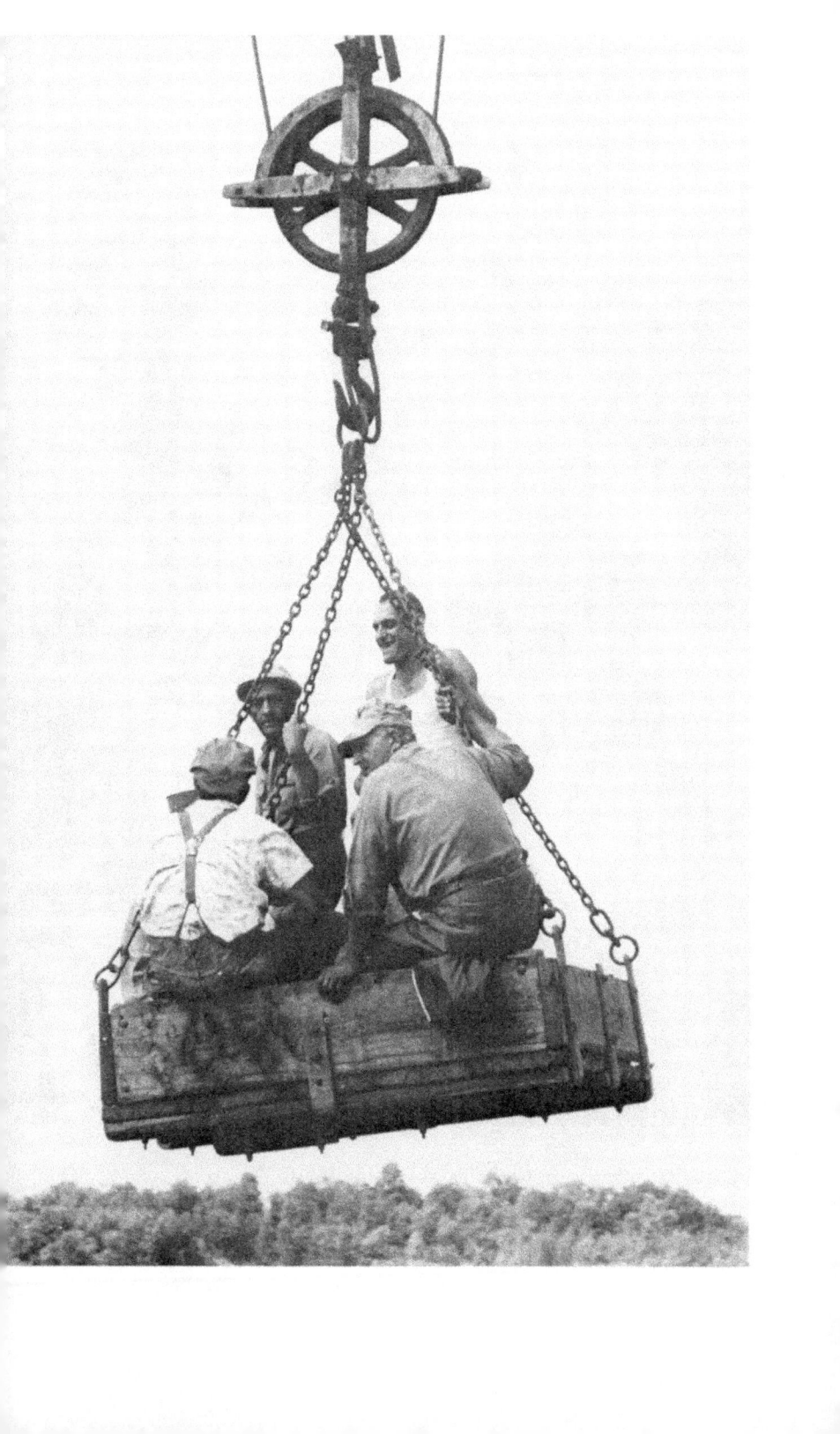

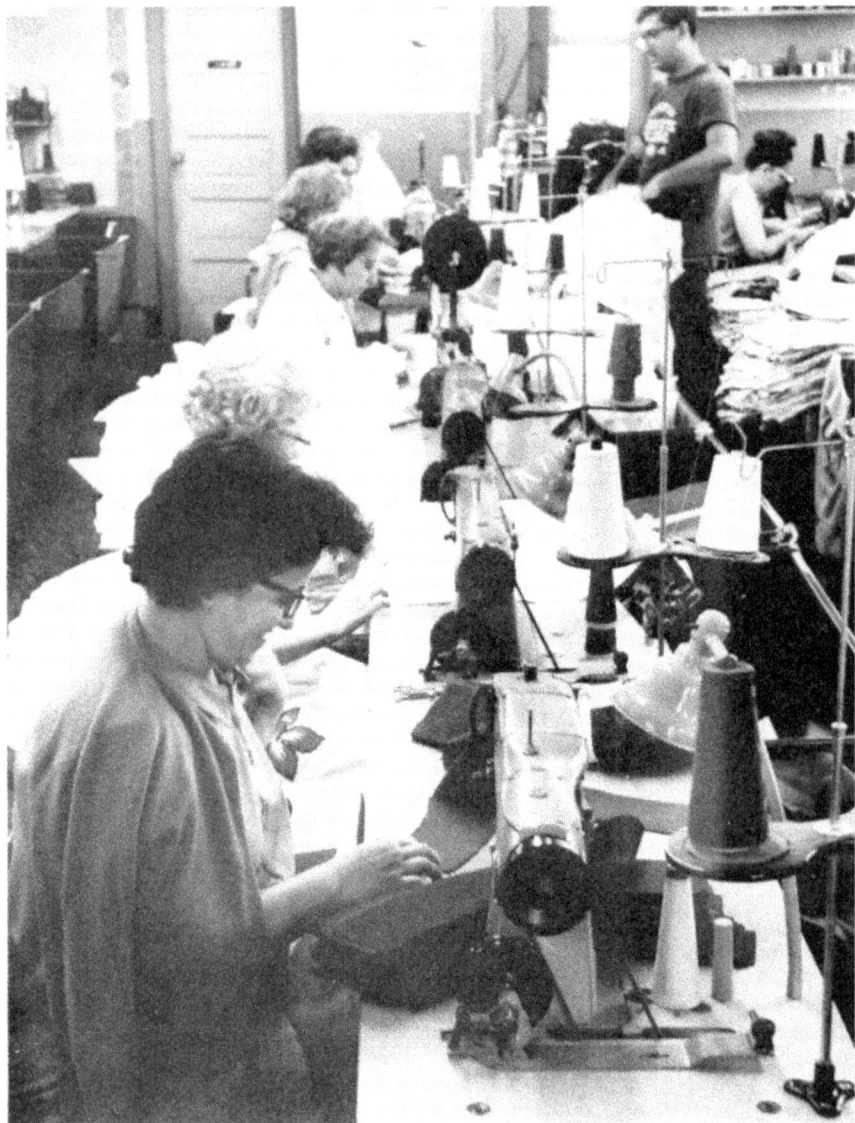

A Roseto blouse factory.

but most work outside the community in cement and steel mills, in other nearby industries, or in road construction as skilled laborers. A few are salesmen, technicians, or proprietors of their own small businesses in or near Roseto. The economy of Roseto is dependent primarily on sixteen small textile factories that finish women's blouses and one paper-box factory. Nearly three quarters of the women in Roseto work in these jointly owned family enterprises. Most of the lawyers, engineers, physicians, dentists, osteopaths, and chiropractors who grew up in Roseto live in Bangor or other nearby towns. Many of the third-generation college-educated youth have moved to other parts of the United States to seek white-collar jobs. Table 10 gives the distribution of Rosetans by sex and occupation.

Our occupational survey yielded the information that, although 87 per cent of all Rosetans had achieved more education than their fathers, only 57 per cent were employed at higher occupational levels than those of their fathers; 29 per cent were at the same occupational level as their fathers; and 14 per cent were at a lower level. Those Rosetans who showed the greatest mobility upward and downward were primarily under age forty-four, while those who were occupationally stable were sixty-five years old and over.

The over-all mean annual gross income for employed males and females in 1966 was $6,300 and $2,450, respectively. Only 12 percent of the men and

TABLE 10

Distribution of Rosetans by Sex and Occupation

Occupational Level*	Males		Females		Totals	
	N =	%	N =	%	N =	%
Executives, professionals	5	1	0	0	5	0.
Proprietors of medium-sized businesses	19	5	14	3	33	4
Administrative personnel; small independent business owners	47	18	18	4	92	10
Clerical and sales workers; technicians	32	8	27	5	59	7
Skilled manual employees	106	26	8	2	114	13
Machine operators; semiskilled employees	111	28	309	62	420	47
Unskilled employees	53	13	4	0.8	57	6
Housewives	0	0	115	23	115	13
Students	3	0.7	0	0	3	0.
Total	403		495		898	

*Hollingshead's occupational levels were used.

4 per cent of the women worked at more than one job, and only 25 per cent of the men and 4 per cent of the women worked more than fifty hours a week in their job. Nevertheless, the combined family incomes of Rosetans enabled them to enjoy a middle-class subsistence in a working-class culture.

Local Schools and Institutions

Few of the older generation had had much schooling, but those between the ages of thirty and forty-five had, for the most part, achieved a high-school education. Despite the ready availability of public education, most Rosetan children still attend the parochial elementary and high schools, and 80 per cent of the high-school graduates attend college. However, only 2 per cent of the population have gone on to graduate or professional schools.

The social life of Roseto revolves around its twenty-two social and civic organizations, the largest of which are the American Legion, the Rod and Gun Club, the Marconi Social Club, the Columbia Fire Company, and the Holy Name Society. Most of these organizations are for men, although some of them have women's auxiliaries. Otherwise, the women are excluded from the clubs except on special occasions. Activities in the clubs consists of bantering, bragging, joking, and Italian drinking games (*morra*) and card games (*briscola* and *tresette*). Men in the fire company cook occasional meals in their club kitchen.

Of the Rosetan men whom we canvassed 81 per cent were members of at least one community organization. Of those who were members 94 per cent were apparently active members. Of the respondents 63 per cent (mainly those over thirty) had expressed the opinion that it was necessary to be active in organizations if one lived in Roseto. Rosetans aged twenty-one to thirty, most of whom were not affiliated with organizations, felt that such membership was not important. Those active in the Marconi Club, the first social organization in the community, were mainly aged sixty-five years and over. Those in the age group fifty-five to sixty-four made up most of the membership of the fire company, while those aged thirty-one to forty-four belonged mainly to the Knights of Columbus. Such community organizations, as they bridged the gap between family activities and solitude, were powerful contributors to Roseto's close-knit character.

The social life of Rosetan women derives from their work in the blouse mills and their participation in church groups, the parent-teachers association, and women's auxiliary groups, as well as from the joint preparation of meals for special family and religious occasions.

Religion

Seventy-five per cent of Rosetans, about twelve hundred people, are Roman Catholic. Of the remaining, 16 per cent are Presbyterian, 2 per cent are Jehovah's Witnesses, approximately 5 per cent belong to other Protestant faiths, and about 2 per cent claim no religious affiliation. Roman Catholics predominate in all age groups, but most Presbyterians and Jehovah's Witnesses are clustered between the ages of forty-four and sixty-four.

The flavor of the community is clearly Roman Catholic. As mentioned earlier, its most important observance each year is the celebration of its patron saint, the Festival of Our Lady of Mount Carmel. A Saturday night carnival precedes the occasion each

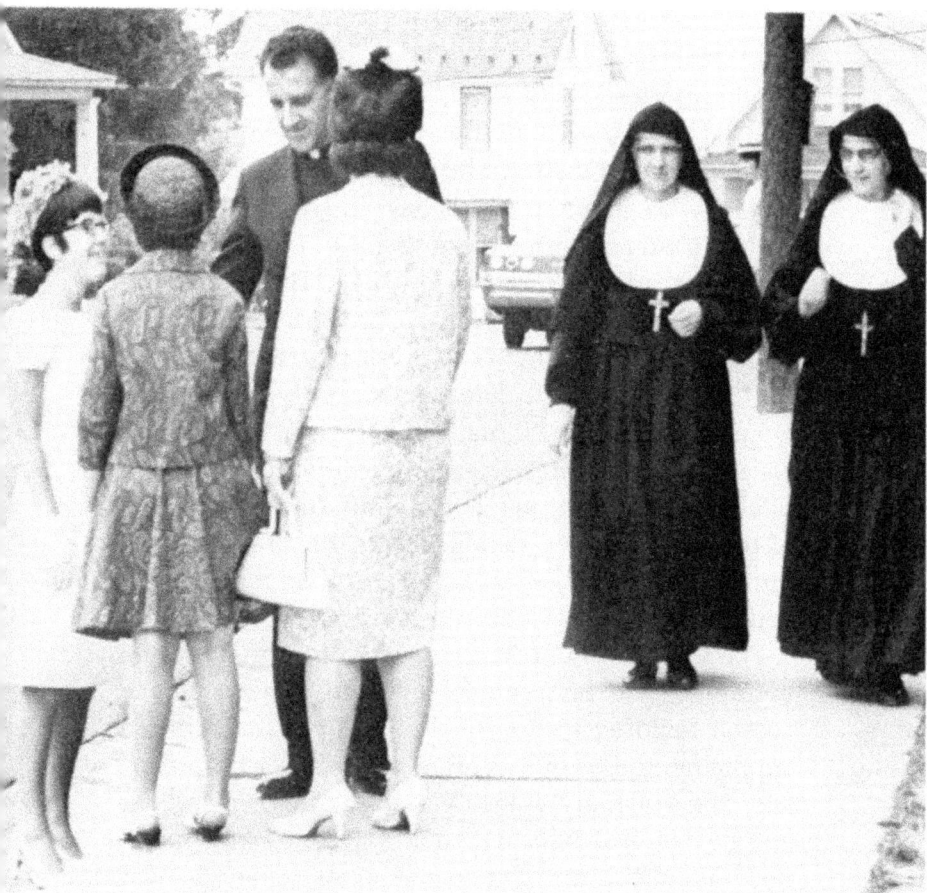

A Sunday afternoon street scene in Roseto.

year during the last week in July. On Sunday after a special mass the statue of the Madonna is brought out of the church and placed on a decorated trailer. The festival queen rides with the statue of the Blessed

Virgin and the Christ child, and her court walks behind. The selection of the queen is a simple and straightforward matter. She is the senior at Pope Pius School who among the girls has shown the most initiative in preparing for the festival. In the procession the priest rides in an open Cadillac. The procession moves down the entire length of Garibaldi Avenue and back to the church. The music is supplied by the Roseto Cornet Band. The men's and women's religious societies, the Mutual Aid Society of Saint Philip Neri and the Sacred Heart Sodality, march separately, and the faithful fall in behind. In the past some of the older women marched barefoot to show their humility and their gratitude for the good fortune that had befallen the Rosetans in America.

The Church of Our Lady of Mount Carmel, on the boundary line between Roseto and Bangor, is the largest building in Roseto. Rosetan parishioners are supplemented by at least an equal number from Bangor. The sanctuary of the church is in Roseto, and the entrance is in Bangor (it is said that one worships in Roseto and tithes in Bangor). A small cemetery with large monuments surrounds the sanctuary. The Presbyterian church, a frame structure with an adjoining manse, stands in the center of town on Garibaldi Avenue. It has about 250 members. The church of the Jehovah's Witnesses, Kingdom Hall, is on the western edge of town. Nearby but outside the city limits of Roseto are two predominantly Italian Episcopal churches. A family's religious affiliation tends to

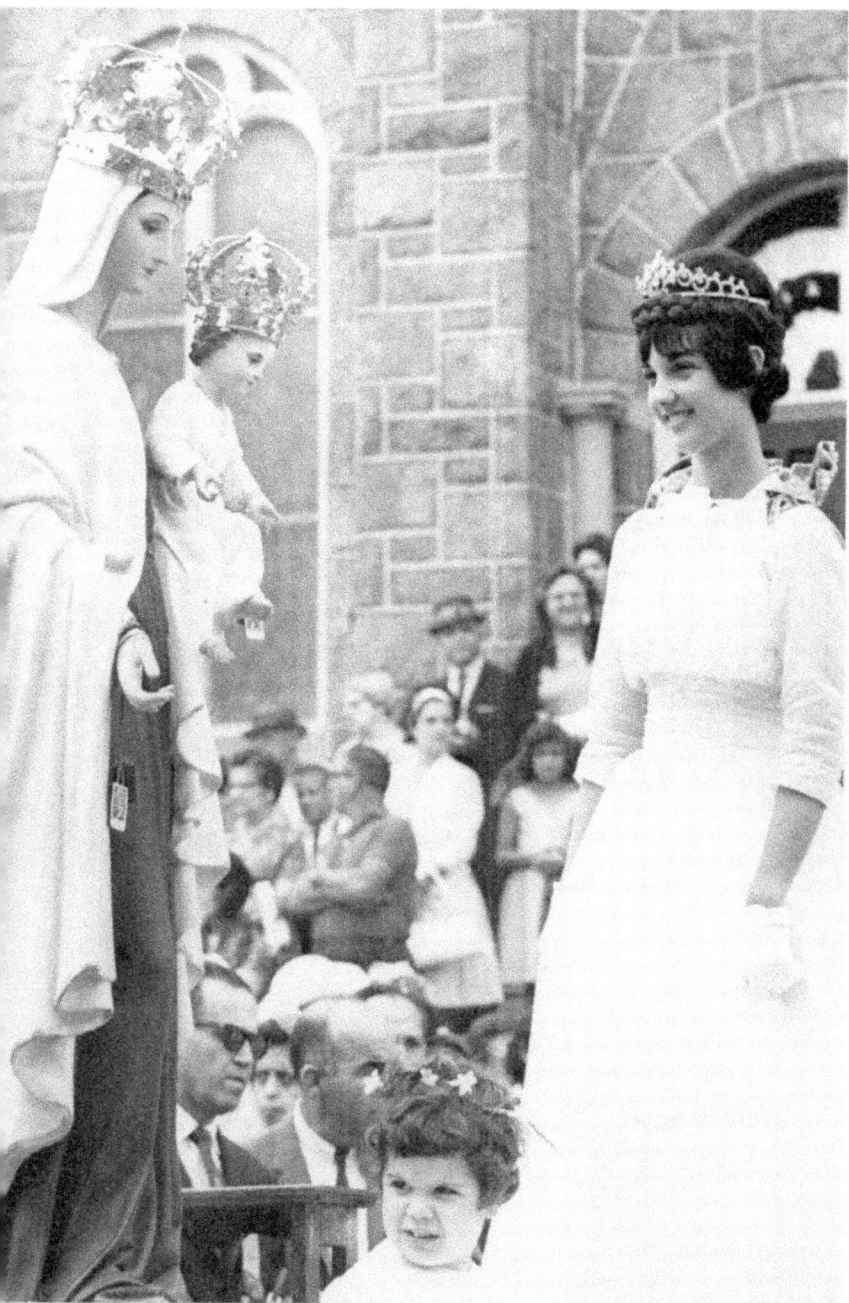

The Queen of the Festival of Our Lady of Mount
Carmel with the statue of the Madonna and Child
(photograph by Steve Schapiro).

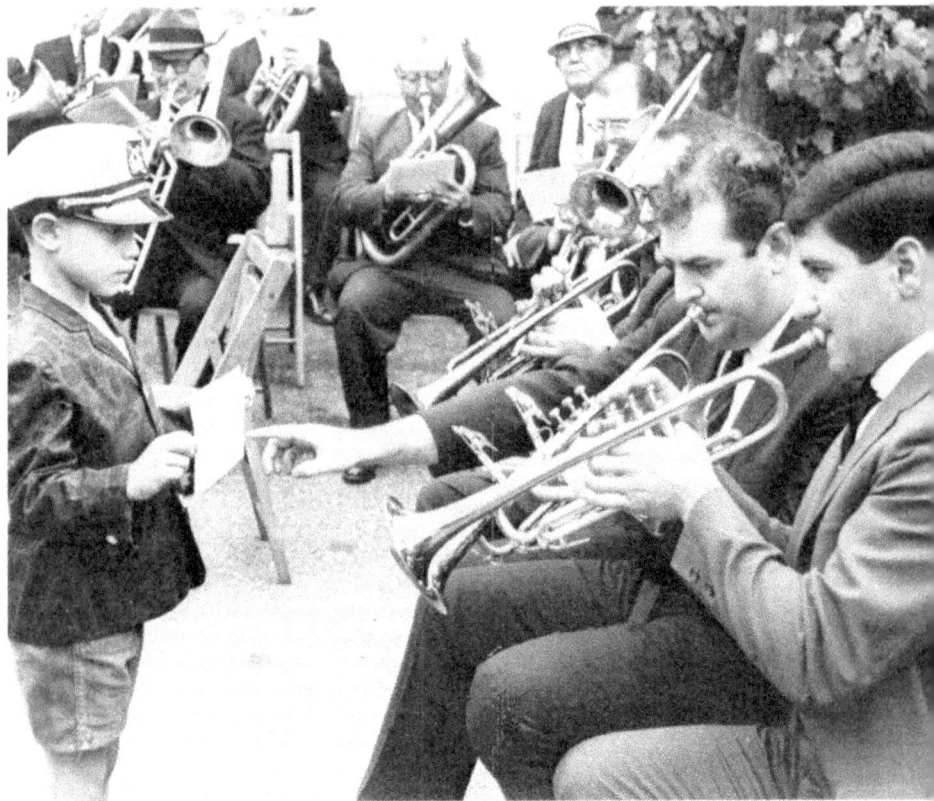

The Roseto Cornet Band rehearsing (photograph by Steve Schapiro).

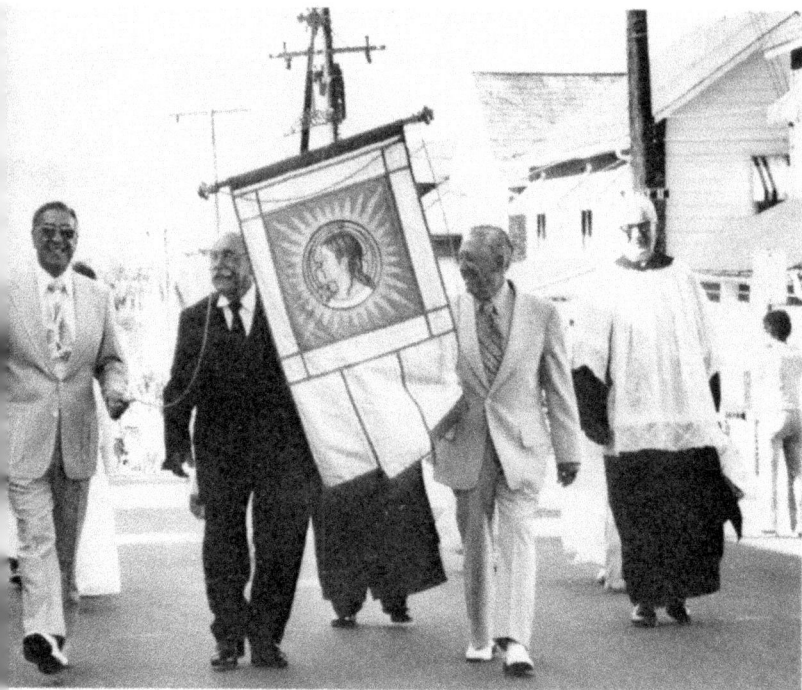

Men carrying the banner of Saint Philip Neri.

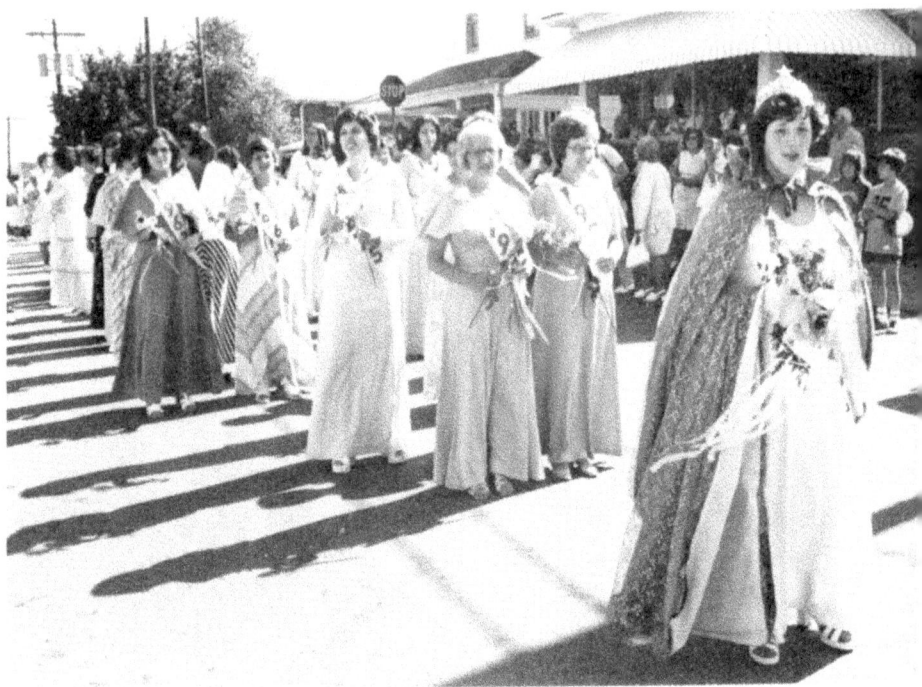

The new Queen leading the former queens of the Festival.

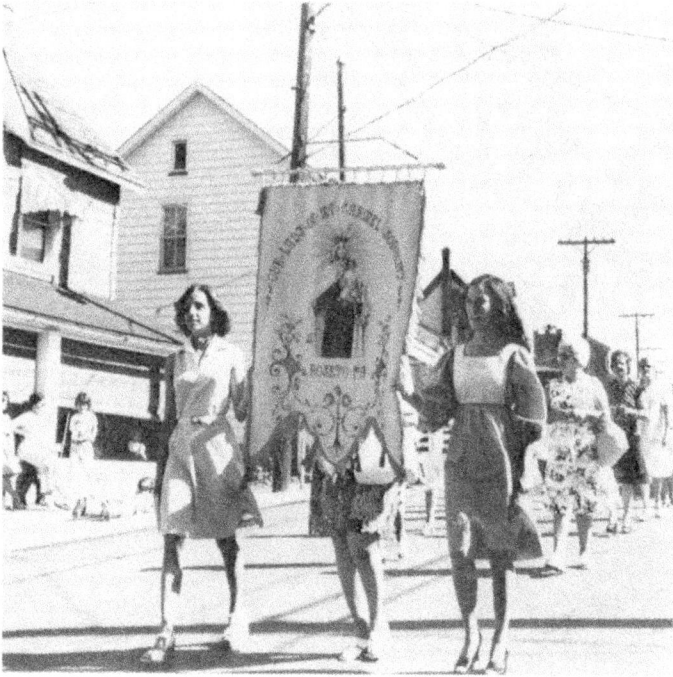

Women carrying the banner of the Sacred Heart
Sodality.

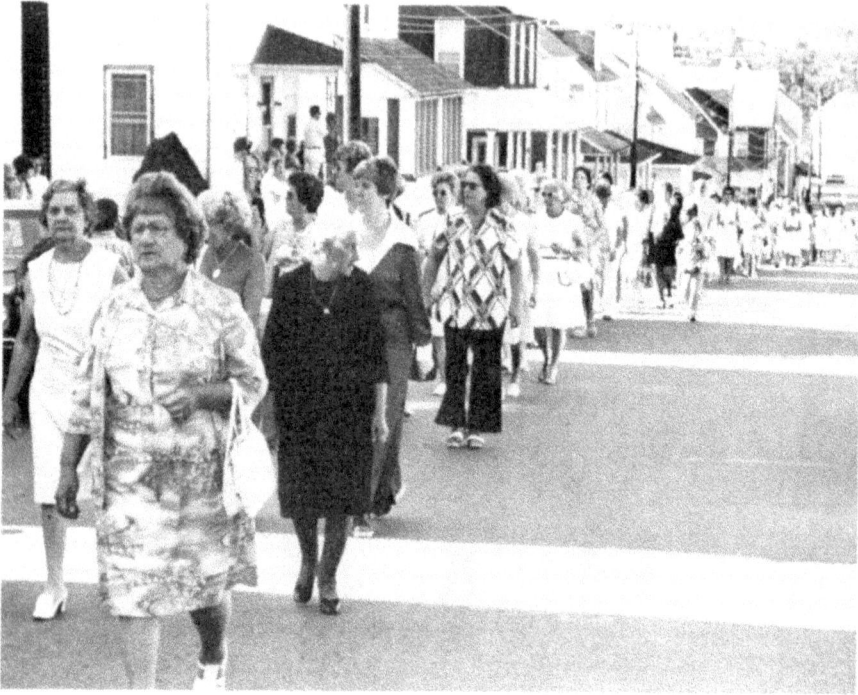

The marchers on Garibaldi Avenue.

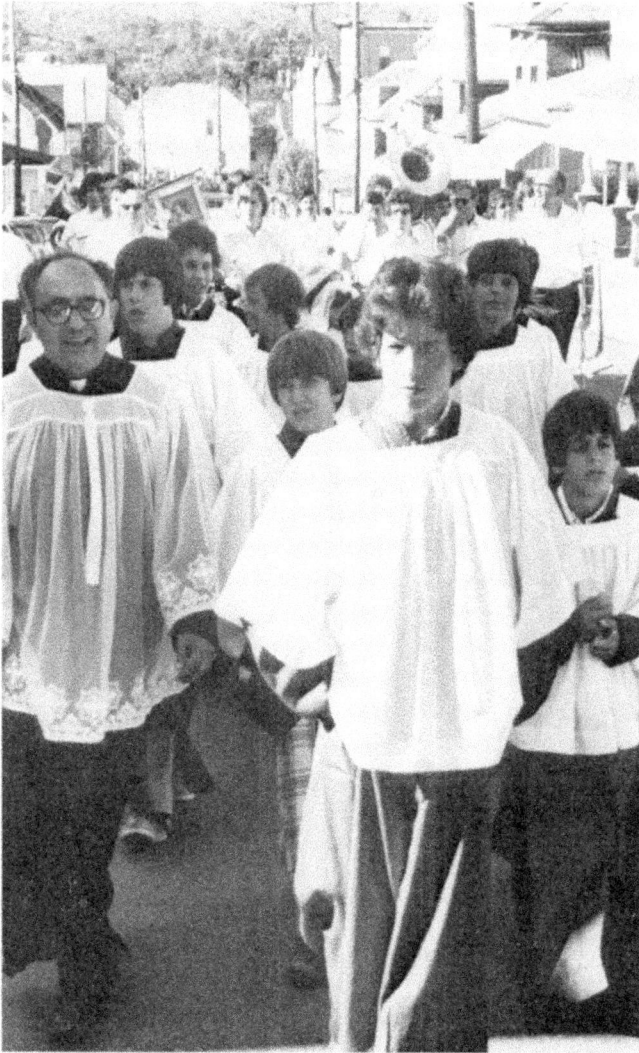

The altar boys.

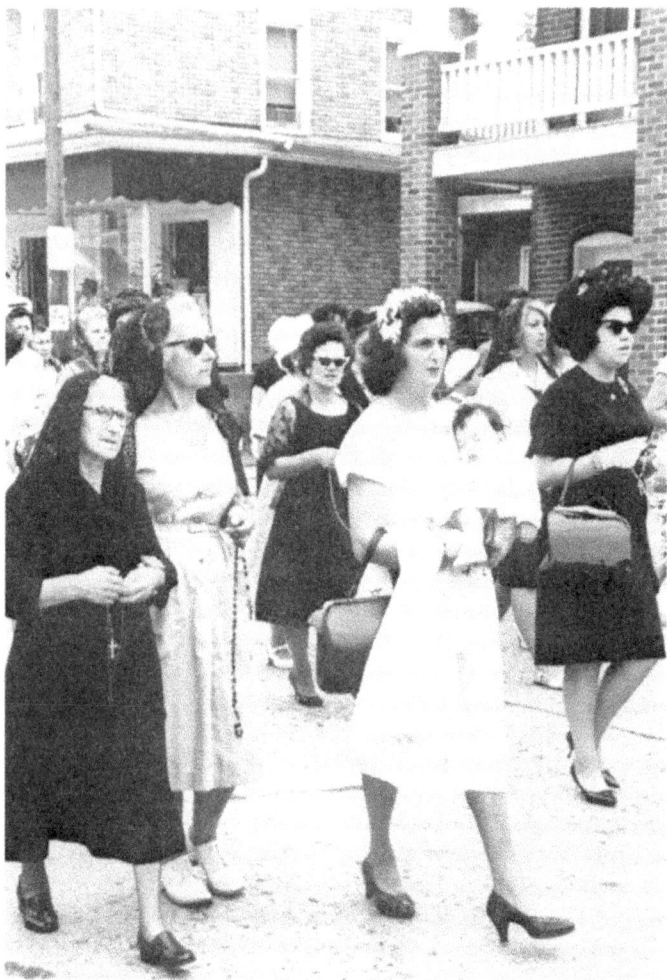

The faithful in procession (photograph by Steve Schapiro).

The Church of Our Lady of Mount Carmel.

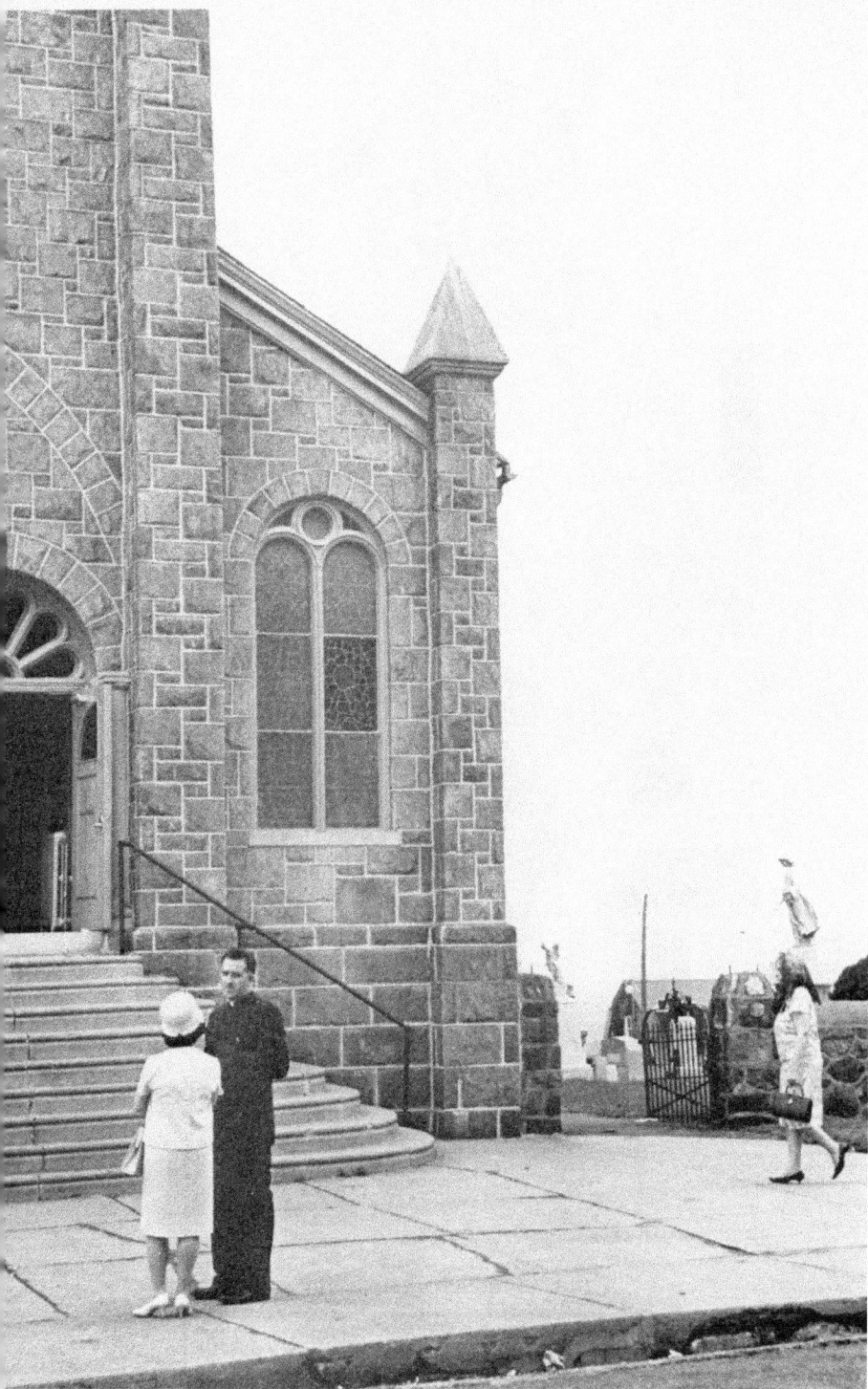

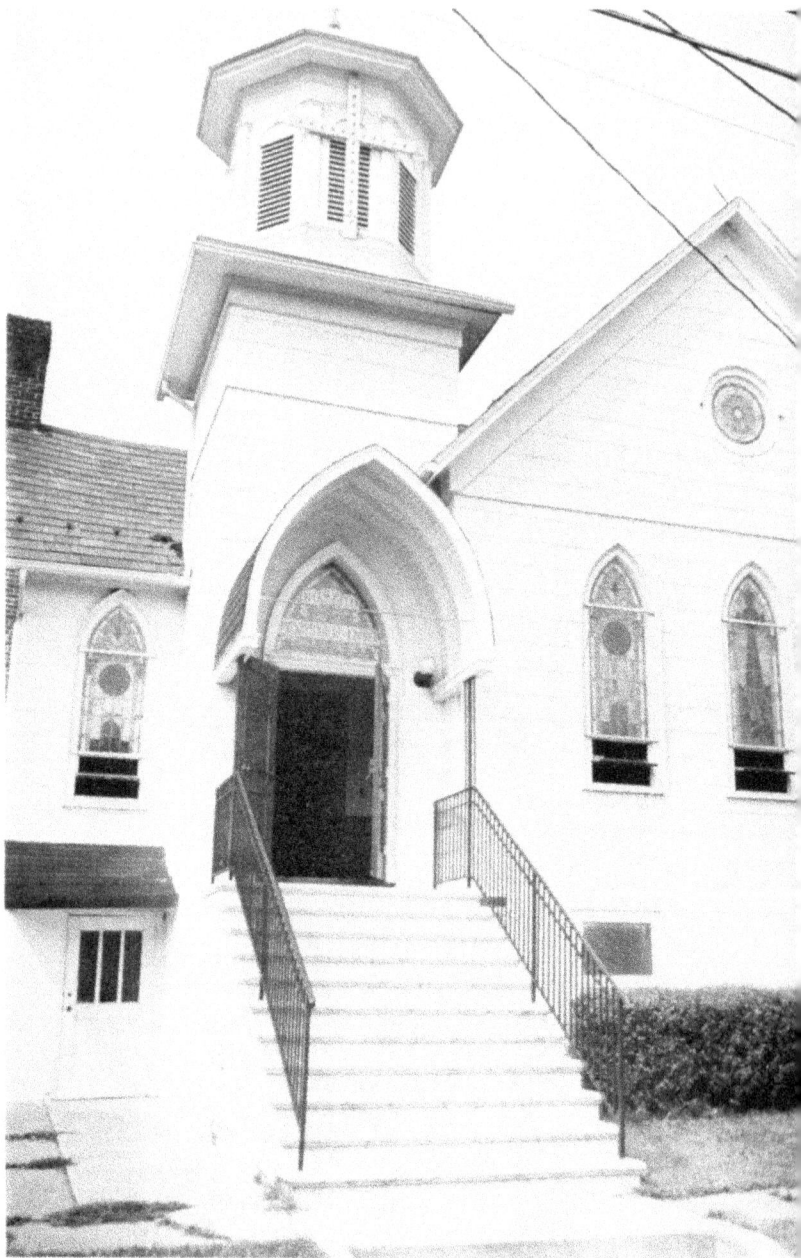

The Old Roseto Presbyterian Church.

coincide roughly with where it lives in Roseto. Most of the Protestants live in the northern section of the town, and the Roman Catholics in the southern section.

Administration and Politics

Since its legal recognition as an independent borough in 1912, Roseto has functioned under a mayor-council form of government. There are 973 registered voters, with an almost equal representation of Democrats and Republicans. Rosetans have given less attention to the political party affilation of a candidate, however, than to his personal characteristics and family ties. Family and clan associations and rivalries are the major factors in town politics. The mayor, therefore, as a political figurehead represents his family in directing the town's activities, and thus his successes and failures reflect upon his extended family. Two recent mayors of the community—young men and political rivals who represented different interest groups—were both from families that originated in Naples, Italy. The political character of the town was reflected in a controversy over a minipark established for the children during a Republican mayorship. It has since been called "Republican Park" by those who viewed it as unnecessary, because a larger public park already existed. The construction of a city sewer system and the assessment of $7.40 a frontage foot from all property owners raised the ire of many against the mayor and council. Political power rests mainly with

the Roman Catholics. Thus the priest plays a significant, if informal, role in community politics, chiefly as
a personal adviser to the mayor.

Social Values

The community also places a high value on economic
success and competitive success of many sorts, even
success in charitable drives. There is a strong tradition of helping one's friends as well as one's family in
Roseto. The success of one who has been helped by
his friend reflects favorably on the helper. Thus the
social emphasis is on interdependence. Luigi Barzini,
who has described such characteristics as typical of
Italians in general, points out that there are vocational
areas where these rules are suspended, such as
medicine, law, and other professions where success
results from greater individual independence, self-
control, and responsibility (1). It is interesting in this
regard that Rosetans who have achieved professional
status do not return to live in the community but
rather settle in Bangor or other communities. Nevertheless, they maintain close family ties. The people of
Roseto are proud of these professionals and identify
them as children from their community who made
good. Outside of maintaining Rosetan family ties,
Rosetan professionals who live in Bangor or elsewhere seem to have rejected the kind of community
life they grew up in, as if to say, "I don't need your
help any longer." This attitude was evident in an

interview with a professional who lived his early life in Roseto and now lives in Bangor.

Frank, a successful dentist, was born in Roseto and lived there until he was eighteen, when he went away to college and dental school. Upon graduation he established an office in Bangor but visited Roseto every Friday to eat spaghetti with his father. He said: "I came from a poor family. My father had a small store in Roseto. I saw my father and brother sacrificing for my education. I couldn't let them down. I owed it to them. A boy has to prove himself to be a champion all the way." He married a Protestant girl of German ancestry. "I wouldn't marry an Italian girl," he said. "Italian mothers are too possessive of their children; you never know when they're yours or theirs." He said that he and his wife lived mainly to themselves. Most of their friends were of Welsh extraction:

I feel accepted in Bangor. We're not as excitable or impulsive as Rosetans. People in Roseto are frugal, economical, but for something that shows, they pay a high price. Some people in Roseto embarrass me; they don't know how to reach out, they're still in a shell; they are jealous, belligerent. In Roseto they help you when you're down. When you're up, they cut you down—they throw stones—if you can withstand it, you're a giant, if you crumble, they have no use for you.

Proper behavior by those Rosetans who have achieved material wealth or occupational prestige requires attention to a delicate balance between ostentation and reserve, ambition and restraint, modesty and dignity, lightheartedness and gravity. The local priest emphasized that when preoccupation with earning money exceeded the unmarked boundary it became a basis for social rejection, irrespective of the standing of the person outside the community. Similarly, a lack of concern for community needs, especially by those who would spend their money on frivolous pleasures, constituted grounds for social exclusion. Rosetan culture thus provided a set of checks and balances to ensure that neither success nor failure got out of hand. Ambition and enhancing one's status were highly valued and expected of the Rosetan male, but overambition was discouraged; the individual achievement of power elicited both fear and resentment from one's fellows. On the other hand, if an individual was not thought to be ambitious or had the wanderlust, the community might point a finger at him as not living up to community standards.

After achieving his goal, a man was usually required to stand a test, that is, to prove to his own people that he was capable of reaching his goal. A demonstration of one's capabilities to outsiders was not sufficient to pass this test, although one might escape the test by living away from the Roseto-Bangor area. The test consisted of the verbal "stone throwing" referred to above. The individual's goal or status was not criticized; rather, the individual himself was the focus of the remarks. The community, having supported him in the achievement of his goal, tested the individual's ability to cope with success. This process was seemingly the final step in preparing the individual to meet the threats and uncertainties he would encounter in his relationship with others in his future life and in assessing the strength of his loyalty to his group. (This testing ordeal resembled that widely practiced by black groups as "the dozens." Often after choosing a leader they will "put him in the dozens," reviling and insulting him for several minutes to test his equanimity, resilience, and good humor.)

During our community survey in 1966, forty-three of those interviewed, or 5 per cent, said that they were "outsiders" in the community. Twenty-five of the forty-three had been born elsewhere. Most were non-Italians who had married Italians born in Roseto. Half of them were Protestant. Their mean age (36.4 years) was younger than the mean age of the community, and they had achieved more years of education (10.7 years). A small number of the non-Italian outsiders had no Italian ties through marriage, worked outside of the community, and did not participate in Rosetan social life or organizations or have close friends or relatives in Roseto.

Social Stratification

During the first five years of our study it was difficult to distinguish, on the basis of dress or behavior, the wealthy from the impecunious in Roseto. Living arrangements (houses and cars) were simple and strikingly similar. Despite the affluence of many, there was no atmosphere of "keeping up with the Joneses" in Roseto, no "putting on the dog." In most families both husbands and wives worked, and virtually all the women did their own housework. Poorer families were quietly provided for, usually by their relatives. The Bangor Department of Public Welfare carried only four Rosetan families on their records during the period 1945 to 1966. All four of them had moved to Roseto from East Bangor and were either non-Italians or were products of ethnically mixed marriages.

We found social distinctions to be more readily identified on the basis of family than income. Descendants of original settlers from Roseto Valfortore enjoyed especially high status. Status could be earned, however, by working hard for the community, by living by the rules and upholding community standards, and especially by achieving a college or professional education. Solid, dependable citizenship; home ownership and maintenance of one's home; regular attendance at church; and generous subscription to charitable and other community causes were the marks of those accorded the greatest respect. Italian Americans who were not Roseto natives were well accepted in the community, but only conditionally until they had learned the English language and demonstrated conformity to local customs and values.

Herbert J. Gans observed four major behavior types

among Italian Americans in Boston's West End (19). He called them *routine seekers, middle-class mobiles, action seekers,* and *maladapted.* We recognized such types in Roseto. The routine seekers were, in our perception, mainly first- and second-generation families who held firmly to Old World traditions and lived by established patterns. Even the food items to be eaten on certain days of the week were clearly prescribed and adhered to. The routine seekers found security and satisfaction in familiar and predictable circumstances. Somewhat younger and, at the time our study began, in much smaller numbers were the middle-class mobiles, who sought "social advancement" in professional education and business contacts outside Roseto. A few of these, especially the more affluent, became action seekers in their inclinations toward entertainment and travel and their more mercenary attitudes. The maladapted, initially very few, were mainly those who had broken away from Rosetan traditions by marrying non-Italians, by spending freely, and by dissociating themselves from formerly close family and community ties. The balance among these social types was to shift in a few years toward a larger proportion of middle-class mobiles and action seekers, as discussed in Chapters 5 and 6.

Throughout the decade of the 1960's the number of first-generation Rosetans declined through death. The second-generation and many of the third-generation Rosetans maintained the routine-seeking point of view for themselves but encouraged their children to enhance their education and thus become middle-class mobiles. We were able to observe evidences of impending social change as early as 1963. The indications came mainly from those under age thirty, from those born after the Great Depression of 1929 to 1934, and especially from teenagers, as discussed in Chapters 5 and 6.

4
Roseto's Neighbors: Bangor and Nazareth

At the time of this study Bangor had a population of
about five thousand. It had been settled as a farming
community by Scotch-Irish immigrants and German
Mennonites (the Pennsylvania Dutch). Part of what
now constitutes the one and one-half square miles of
the borough of Bangor was earlier known as Howell
Town and the rest as Cricktown, a name thought to
have derived from the many small creeks in the area.
As the population increased, what is now the central
portion of Bangor was called New Village, while the
older portion became known as Uttsville. Slate deposits, discovered at about the time of the Civil War,
attracted an immigration of Welshmen. One such
pioneer slater, Robert M. Jones, suggested that the
community be named after his home, Bangor, a

slate-mining community in northwest Wales. The new town was incorporated in 1873, and Jones became the first chief burgess.

Bangor was primarily an agricultural community until the early 1880's, when the income from the English- and Welsh-owned slate quarries and small businesses in the area outstripped the farming income of the Pennsylvania Dutch. Then the Welsh ethnic character was gradually lost as other immigrants came to work in the slate quarries.

Around 1912 three glove-manufacturing plants were established in Bangor, and in 1919 and 1920 the Kaiser Silk Company bought the plants, consolidated them, and began producing full-fashioned hosiery. The Kaiser plant employed about fifteen hundred people and operated twenty-four hours a day, becoming one of the largest producers of hosiery in the United States. Bangor prospered until the depression of the late 1920's and early 1930's, when the First National Bank in Roseto and the Bangor Trust Company, after losing an estimated three million dollars, closed their doors, never to reopen. The bank failures contributed to the loss of the Kaiser plant, which (because nylon was rapidly displacing silk in the manufacture of women's stockings) was moved in the 1940's to South Carolina, where production costs were lower than in Pennsylvania. Kaiser also established plants in Japan, where the company could produce silk hosiery at one-tenth the cost of manufacture in Bangor.

Those events were paralleled by changes in the slate industry. The twenty slate quarries in the area were threatened by competition from asbestos roof shingles and a consequent decrease in demand for slate. Moreover, it was becoming increasingly difficult to recruit young men to work for low wages in the quarries. The Flory Manufacturing Company, a foundry that manufactured hoists for the slate industry, failed in the 1930's.

One bright spot in the gloomy economic picture was the formation of the Blueridge Textile Company in 1937. It prospered so well that by the end of World War II the expanding plant instituted a profit-sharing plan for employees. In addition, the Slate Belt Industrial Corporation was formed in the 1950's to attract industry to the area, and local bankers made contributions to bring Hires Products, producers of light metal and auto parts, to the area in 1958. Hires employed about two hundred people. Nevertheless, the economy continued to decline while the Bangor Chamber of Commerce insisted that heavy industry pay high wages, and only one of the two local banks actively supported industrial mortgages. The older wealthy people of the community took no part in civic groups. Clubs were used for social purposes rather than to help the town progress. Bangor men began to seek work in Easton and Bethlehem with Ingersol Rand, Bethlehem Steel, and the Pennsylvania Pump and Compressor Company. Thus Bangor became a bedroom community where people lived and slept but worked elsewhere. Bangor also lost population because college graduates did not return to live and work in the community.

The economic stagnation of the community was intimately tied to its social and ethnic structure. The thirty to fifty families whose assets were valued at $100,000 or more lacked public spirit, and few of them assumed leadership roles. Most wanted to maintain the status quo and were politically inactive. The community leaders were primarily the executives of Bangor banks and industries and the officers of local social clubs. A mayor's committee to "uplift" the town failed because of political rivalry. The English were described as "clannish," and the English-Welsh and Pennsylvania Germans as a "proud group" who "stand on their own feet." As one respondent said, "If I had to depend on the people of Bangor for business there wouldn't be any—people pull for themselves here." Another said, "People keep their problems to themselves here—Protestants figure out things independently."

The rivalry of the several ethnic groups has kept the town of Bangor segmented throughout its history, although the arrival of large numbers of Italians in Bangor around 1900 caused the English, Welsh, and Germans to consolidate to some extent. Italians were excluded from the Masonic Lodge, social clubs, and political office until the 1960's and 1970's. Only in recent years have Italians been elected to community posts. Nevertheless, nearly 25 per cent of Bangorians are Italian, most of whom live in the second and fourth wards in north and northwest Bangor, adjacent to Roseto.

Although 33 per cent of Bangor's population of slightly over five thousand is Roman Catholic, there is only one Catholic church. There are eight Protestant churches (Methodist, Presbyterian, Lutheran, Dutch Reformed, and Moravian), each established during a different ethnic immigration. None has a really strong or cohesive congregation. One minister said, "We have no membership directory—there is a looseness in the organization of the church, an 'I don't care' attitude about neighbors." He also related a lack of interest in the summer Bible school and covered-dish dinners. Another minister said that only 40 to 60 per cent of his members are regular church attenders. "We don't have involvement—they don't want to get involved even on Sunday mornings—but they resent it very much if they are told that their membership had lapsed, because they want it to be known when they die that they belong to a church." In addition, he stated, "It's heartbreaking organizational work." Several ministers longingly noted the "sense of commitment the Catholic Church requires, especially of the Italians."

The history of Nazareth began in central Europe, where in the fifteenth century the followers of John Huss formed a small group known as the Unitas Fratrum, Fratres Bohemiae now known as the Moravians.

During the following three centuries religious perse-
cution drove the Moravians to Protestant centers in
Poland and Germany. Early in the eighteenth century
they were offered refuge in Germany on the estate of
Count Nicholas Ludwig von Zinzendorf, a Lutheran
and a benefactor of other Protestant sects. Among
those other sects were the followers of Kaspar
Schwenkfeld, a German nobleman of Silesia, whose
unorthodox views elicited hostility both from
Catholics and from other Protestants (27).

The banishment of the Schwenkfelders from
Saxony in 1733 led Zinzendorf to organize their departure to Georgia in the United States, where they
had been offered a tract of land and free passage by
James Oglethorpe. On the way the Schwenkfelders
stopped over in Holland. While there they learned
that Oglethorpe had failed to produce the needed
travel funds. Instead, therefore, some of them em-
barked for Pennsylvania, to which they had also been
offered free passage. The freedom of religion in
Pennsylvania and the pacifism of the Quakers made
William Penn's colony attractive to them, and also to
other Moravians who had originally emigrated to
Georgia. In 1740 the Moravians settled the Barony of
Nazareth, Pennsylvania, a five thousand-acre tract of
land bought by George Whitefield, a Methodist missionary, along the fork of the Delaware and Lehigh
rivers (32, 41).

Whitefield, who had come to Pennsylvania from
Georgia, hoped to establish a free school for Negro

children and a village for destitute Englishmen. He appointed Peter Boehler, the leader of one of the groups of Moravians, to construct the school. Conflicts soon arose between Whitefield and Boehler over religious views, and the Methodist ordered the Moravians to leave. Thereupon they bought five hundred acres of land nearby at the present site of Bethlehem. Soon after, Whitefield's financial backer died, forcing him to abandon his plan for the Negro school. He sold the barony to the Moravians and returned to England.

The Moravians set about building houses at intervals between Bethlehem and Nazareth where missionaries and traveling brethren could seek refuge. Indians living at Wilagamika, a village on the Nazareth tract, did not recognize the claims of the Moravians. Zinzendorf, who was working among the Creek and Cherokee Indians near Savannah, Georgia, was summoned to manage the dispute. Unsuccessful in negotiation, he found it necessary to repurchase the land inhabited by the Indians to ensure their departure. Zinzendorf thereupon took over as leader of the Nazareth and Bethlehem community. He planned to make Nazareth the central church village and Bethlehem the school center. Since missionary work was of primary concern to Zinzendorf, he assigned groups of Moravians to work among the Indians and whites as missionaries. Zinzendorf was hoping to draw the Pennsylvania Dutch Protestant churches and Quakers together in a union. The

Lutheran and Reformed churches, both in need of clergymen, responded favorably, but the Mennonites, Dunkards, and Ephrata—suspicious of Zinzendorf's intentions—declined. Alarmed at Zinzendorf's actions, the Lutheran and Reformed church hierarchies in Europe soon sent ministers to save their congregations.

Zinzendorf organized the communal system, called the General Economy, at both Bethlehem and Nazareth. No one was paid wages. Instead, everyone became part of one household and worked for the good of the whole. The church owned all the land, buildings, and tools. Bishop Spangenburg and his wife headed the General Economy, presiding over the committees that managed the details of government. Both the communities were self-sufficient. Bethlehem became the center of trade and industry, while Nazareth remained an agricultural community.

Under the General Economy each person received the necessities of life and also free education, medical care, and care in old age. There was social equality despite the presence of several noblemen, who helped establish high standards of education, fine arts, music, and gracious living.

Several disasters plagued the communities, however, including attacks from hostile Indians and smallpox epidemics. The European church was exerting restrictive control, and finally with the departure of the original leaders, Spangenberg and Boehler, the old order began to change. Zinzendorf died in 1756, leaving the church more than one million dollars in debt. The communities paid the debt in full, but by 1762 the General Economy had been abrogated, and the privilege of private lease of land or business was instituted.

The communities were divided into age groups called choirs, each living separately. As soon as the children were old enough to be separated from their mothers, they were placed in the nursery to be cared for by widows and single and married women who were not strong enough for other work. There were also choirs for single sisters, single brethren, widows, and married sisters and brethren. Each choir had its own house and distinctive way of life.

Dress was also regulated. The women dressed in plain gray or brown dresses with white caps tied with bows of different colors (*Schneppelhauben*): red bows for little girls, rose for older girls, pink for single women, blue for married women, and white for widows. Men wore broadbrimmed hats, dark coats without lapels, and knee britches.

Before marriage boys and girls grew up separately, lived separately, sat on separate sides of the church, and were buried separately. With the belief that marriage is a lottery, man was thought to be assured of divine guidance in choosing a wife. The caretakers of single sisters and brethren arranged marriage by lot. If they were not satisfied, brethren could ask the authorities to choose again or could go to another community and try their luck in selecting a marriage partner. The girl was under no compulsion to marry her match, but so much importance was attached to the divine element that she often let herself be guided by the lot.

Love feasts, characteristic of the Moravian church since 1727, were an important part of the life of the Nazareth settlement, and they are still a church ceremony today. The love feast is primarily a song service opened with prayer and followed by the congregation's partaking of food and drink as a sign of their unity and equality. There is no rule about the food to be offered at love feasts as long as it is simple and easily distributed. It is not consecrated as are the elements in the Communion. Nowadays the drink may be coffee, tea, or lemonade. Mugs from a tray brought along the aisle are passed from hand to hand in the pew, and a slightly sweetened bun is usually served from baskets. Children and members of any denomination may participate, but the servers, or *dieners*, must be "born Moravians." The men usually distribute the drink, and the women the basket of bread. Today love feasts, originally established to build morale and offset the hard pioneer life, can be held during church festivals or anniversaries or at any time there is a desire to stress oneness and brotherhood.

The early Moravians were very enterprising. They owned ships that plied the Atlantic between Europe and America. In Bethlehem they established the first public waterworks, fire-fighting equipment, and apothecary shops in America. The first symphony orchestra in the United States was established in the Nazareth-Bethlehem enclave, and both choral music and brass instrumental music have been a notable part of Moravian culture. Trombone choirs customarily announced the death of a member of the community. The children were taught to sing and play musical instruments to accompany ordinary daily work. Each work group sang its own distinctive songs. The musical tradition has been kept alive. Today the yearly presentation by the Bach choir of the B-Minor Mass is a major artistic event attended by visitors from all over the world. The choir also performs periodically in New York City and in European capitals.

Despite its considerable enlightenment, the rigid, restricted character of the Moravian community hampered its adaptation to the evolving American society. Following the abandonment of the General Economy, and especially from 1765 to 1774, Nazareth underwent a period of marked social readjustment. The population dwindled from 351 in 1764 to 251 in 1774. Many visitors began to arrive from other parts of the United States and Europe. A "New Nazareth" began to evolve. Private capitalism spread. Conferences were held to survey the construction of streets, brethren began choosing sites for private homes, and a day school for girls was opened.

The urgent need of the American rebels for firearms prompted the establishment of a gun factory, but because of the pacifism of the Moravians the

factory had to be moved outside the settlement. Although Bethlehem and Nazareth refused to participate in the Revolutionary War, they manufactured
guns for the war and provided food, shelter, and a
hospital for the Continental Army and for British
prisoners. But the war had measurable effects on the
barony, which had grown narrow, timid, conservative, and out of step with the growing American Re-
public. Women had changed to English garments and
had become concerned with food and social affairs
rather than manual work. The single brethren's
house was abandoned in 1814. Some of the single
men migrated to Wachovia and Lititz, North
Carolina. Others changed congregations, a few left
the congregation altogether, some entered Indian
mission work, and others simply moved elsewhere
within the barony. By 1818 the practice of marriage by
lottery had been abandoned. Nevertheless, the community continued as a strictly Moravian enclave, although it was receiving fewer immigrants each year
from abroad.

The heart of Moravian culture lay in the development of education. A school for boys, Nazareth Hall,
was established in 1743. The hall later became a mili-
tary academy and survived until 1779, when it was
closed because of financial problems, the uncertainties of the Revolution, and paucity of residents. In
1785, however, old Nazareth Hall was reopened as a
"pay school" for boys. At the same time a girls school
was established in the Sisters House. The boys

school, including boys from Bethlehem, eventually became a *paedegogium,* or boarding school, and imported most of its faculty from German universities. By 1808 it was attracting pupils from elsewhere on the east coast and even from Europe. A theological seminary was established in 1819 in the home of the former principal of Nazareth Hall. Later the provincial synod founded Moravian College in connection with the seminary. By mid-century, however, financial problems forced the closing of Nazareth Hall again. The seminary and Moravian College were then moved to Bethlehem.

By 1855 the depletion of population in Nazareth, especially the loss of the young people, and the weakening of the economy had prompted the Moravian Overseers Committee to sign an agreement providing for a division of property, bringing to an end more than a hundred years of closed church control. Membership in the church and town was now no longer a requirement to own property in Nazareth. The settlements were opened up. In 1857 the Moravian church in America achieved independence of the European church. By this time Pennsylvanians of German peasant ancestry were flocking into Nazareth. The newcomers established two large churches, the Lutheran and the Reformed, and soon outnumbered the Moravians. The coming of the railroads, the influx of European immigrants, and the need for labor transformed Nazareth into a flourishing industrial center. About 1900, Italians from

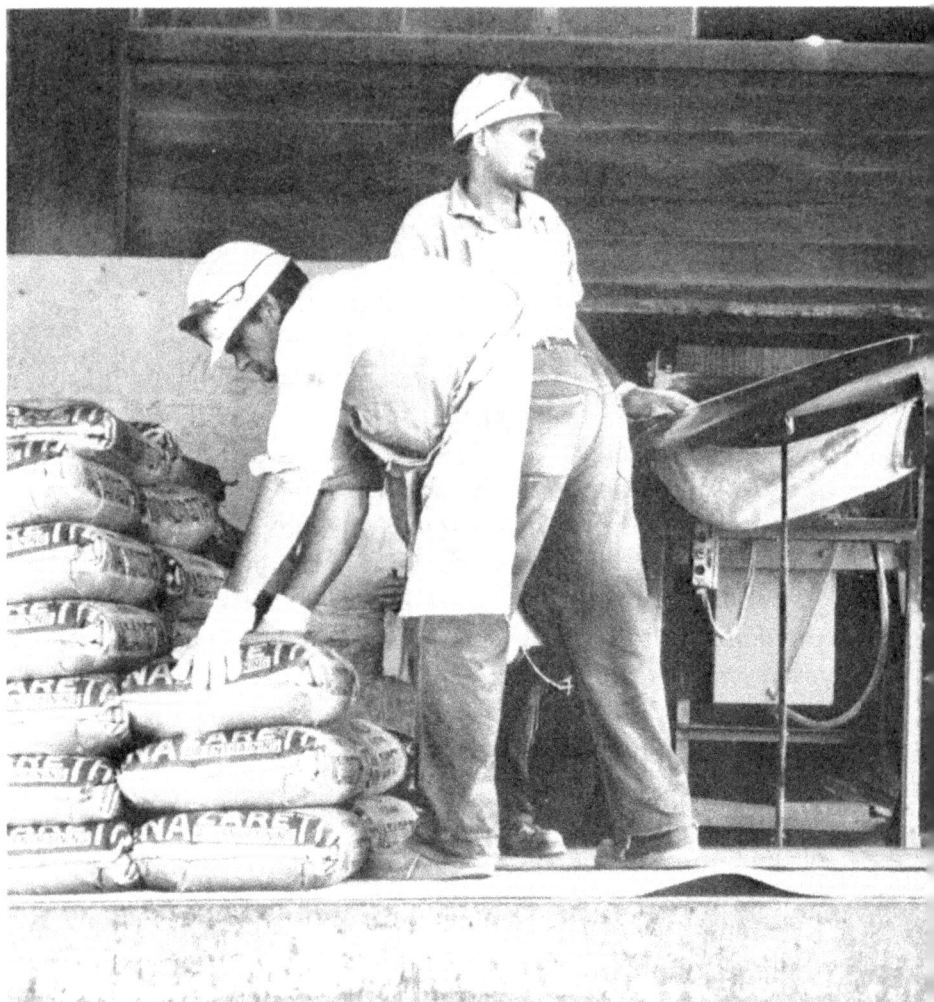

Piling Nazareth cement.

Naples, Trieste, and Sicily, and Poles, Austrians, Hungarians, Yugoslavians, and Czechoslovakians arrived to work in the cement and steel industries. In 1908 a Catholic church was established to serve many of these eastern and southern European immigrants.

Despite its cosmopolitan nature Nazareth maintained a considerable degree of ethnic segregation. The town was geographically divided according to ethnic background. The Italians lived in the south end of town, and the Germans, Austrians, Poles, and Hungarians in the west end. The various ethnic groups lived in red shanties and cement homes provided by the industries for which they worked. The Moravians managed to maintain their higher social status, distinguishing themselves from the less-cultivated Pennsylvania Dutch, who spoke "impure" German. The remnants of these earlier ethnic and religious attitudes are evident in Nazareth today.

Although now outnumbered by the Pennsylvania Dutch, the Moravians continue at the top of the social scale. Those of German extraction comprise about 70 per cent of the population. The English and Welsh comprise about 10 per cent, Italians 5 per cent, and Poles, Austrians, Hungarians, Yugoslavs, Czechoslovakians, Ukranians, French, Spaniards, Swiss, Dutch, Scots, and Irish the remaining 15 per cent. About 77 per cent of the residents are of native parentage, 16 per cent are of foreign or mixed parentage, and 7 per cent are foreign-born. Protestants make up 70 per cent of the population; Roman Catholics, 20 per cent. The largest Protestant denominations are the Lutheran and the Reformed, although six other Protestant denominations are represented (Nazarene, Bible Fellowship, Jehovah Witness, Evangelical, Mennonite, and Moravian). The Jehovah's Witnesses were formed in 1960 by a group of dissenters from the Roseto Jehovah's Witnesses.

As of this writing Nazareth is a prosperous community of 6,208 inhabitants. It is situated on a ridge of solid lime rock five hundred feet above sea level and is the center of a Portland Cement manufacturing region. There are three large cement plants within the borough limits and three just outside. Other industries include the C. F. Martin Company, manufacturer of world-famous guitars, ukuleles, and mandolins since 1831. There are also factories for children's underwear, paper bags and boxes, plastics, steel fabrication, and alfalfa dehydration. Most of the men are employed in Nazareth's twenty-six industries. About 40 per cent of the women in the community are employed.

The complexion of Nazareth has changed greatly since its rapid period of growth between 1900 and 1930. The traditional emphasis on education and culture weakened as Nazareth became a multiethnic industrial community. Indeed, today the educational achievement of its residents is lower than the mean of its school district, the Lehigh Valley region, and of the state and the nation. Only 28 per cent of the residents have completed high school or had additional

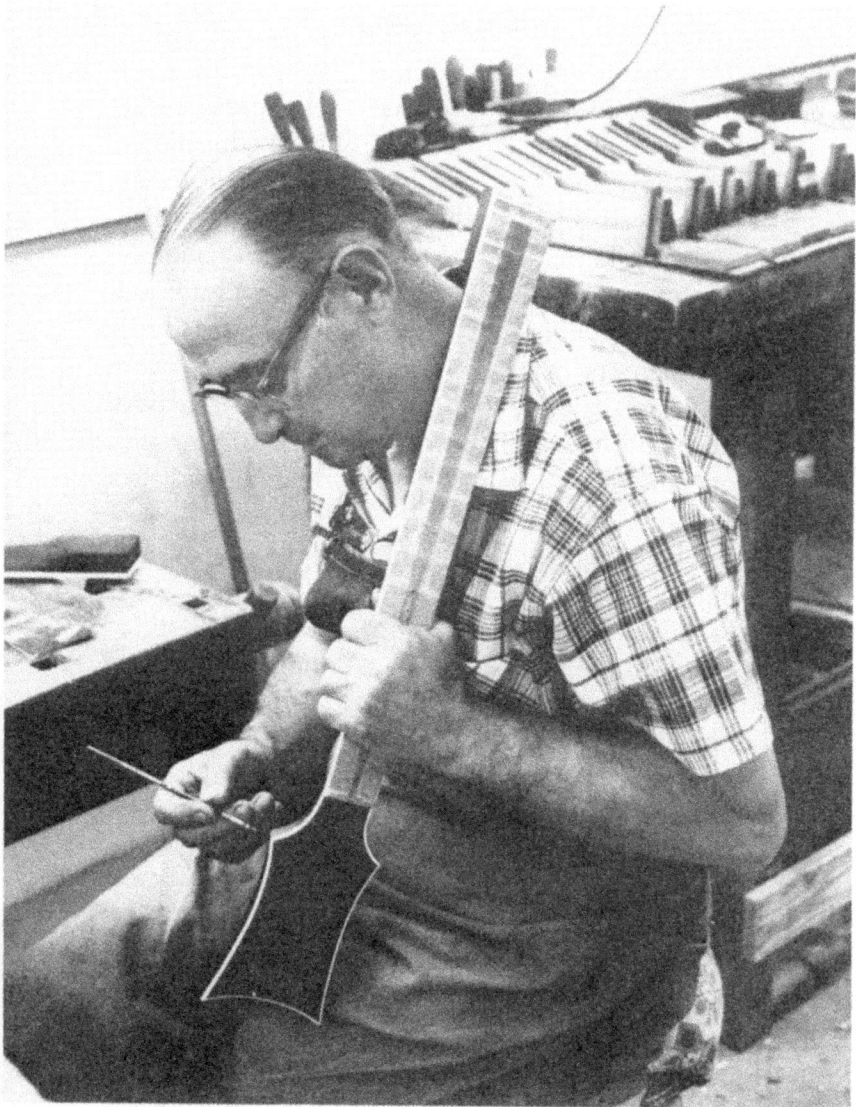

Precision work in the C. F. Martin guitar factory in
Nazareth.

training. The median educational level in present-day Nazareth is 8.8 years. This radical shift in educational balance came about partly because educated young people moved away as elderly people of German peasant background moved in. Consequently Nazareth has a lower percentage of young adults and a higher percentage of middle-aged and elderly people than the rest of the county, the state, and nation. Since 1960 the total population has decreased by 5 per cent, primarily because of the declining importance of cement in the national market and also because the large landholdings of the cement companies had restricted the earlier growth of the borough.

Despite the major social changes, Nazareth is still a prestige address for people of German lineage. As befits the legend that Germans do not flaunt their wealth but are thrifty, hardworking, and conservative, the overt display of wealth is frowned upon by the older residents, although the younger ones have begun to build elaborate homes in the wooded, hilly fringes of the city. A conspicuous neatness pervades the city, which was laid out according to a carefully ordered plan.

The clubs, committees, and social cliques regulate their memberships strictly according to religious and ethnic identification, and social acceptance is difficult for newcomers. To be prominent in the "old days" one had to be an active "born" member of the Moravian church, a property owner, and a partici-

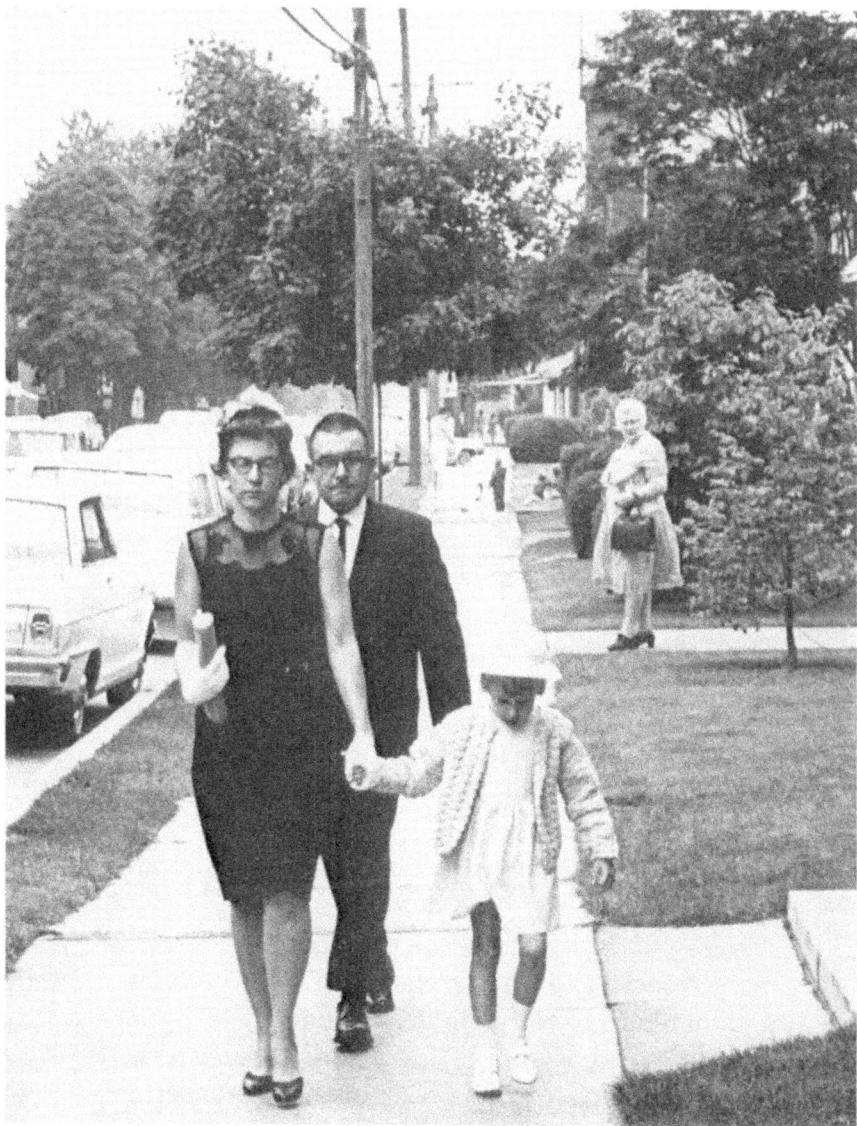

A Sunday street scene in Nazareth.

pant in civic organizations. There are two Moravian churches, one in the center of Nazareth, "the prestige church," and another in the country. Both are stratified along class lines. There are further class distinctions among the other Protestant groups. Although today, for the most part, the old social criteria still apply, there have been some important shifts in the social hierarchy. Teachers and school principals, who once enjoyed high social status and were looked to for leadership in Nazareth's early history, have lost their influence in community affairs. The key positions in the power structure of present-day Nazareth are occupied by the leaders of the steel and cement industries, physicians, lawyers, and bankers.

Nazareth together with its sister city, Bethlehem, was settled in the early 1740's by religious refugees, Moravians from southern Germany. These settlers, better educated and more cultivated than most of their American pioneer neighbors, established a cultured and prosperous community early based on agriculture and ultimately built on the steel and cement industries.

Nazareth in recent years has been undergoing marked social and cultural change. College graduates seldom return to Nazareth to live. Limited job opportunities have encouraged the young people to seek work elsewhere. With the drain of young adults from the population, Nazareth is becoming a community of older people. Although the Moravians have be-

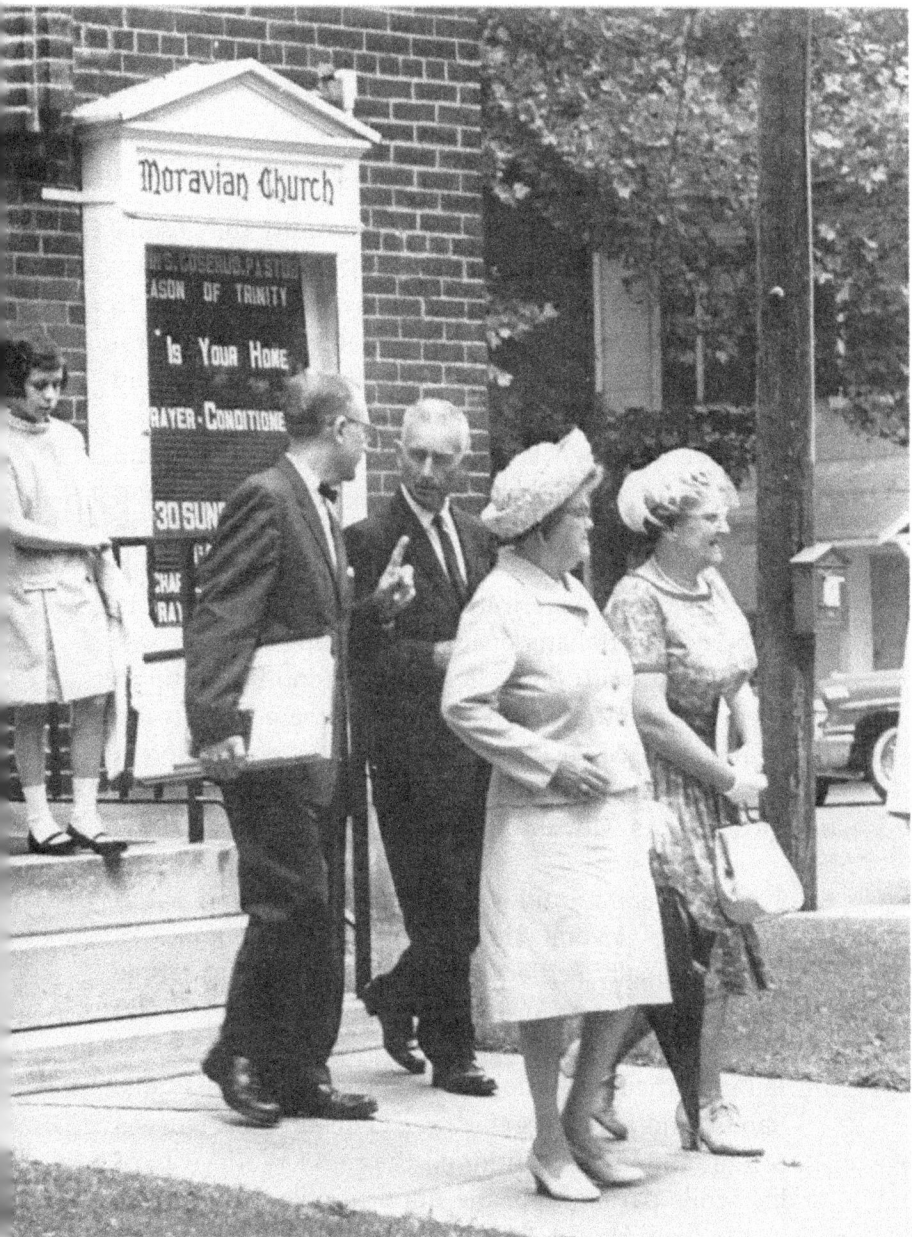

After services in the Moravian Church in Nazareth.

come a minority group in the community they established, they retain their position at the top of the social structure. The historic exclusiveness of Nazareth has lessened as individuals from other ethnic and religious groups have moved into the community and prospered. Community cohesion and family solidarity have loosened considerably as competition and the pace of life have quickened. Since Bangor and Nazareth, like most other industrial communities in the United States, have acquired a substantial proportion of Italian-American citizens, we were able to compare the Italians of Roseto residing in their own community with those living as a minority group in each of the other towns. Thus we were able in the health surveys to compare not only the population at large but also the Italian portion of the population of those towns with the Italians of Roseto.

The three communities of Roseto, Bangor and Nazareth share several characteristics in common. All were originally settled by Europeans seeking refuge from the economic or religious constraints of the Old World. Each began as closed ethnic communities, retaining their traditional ethnic beliefs, customs, habits, and social organization. For different lengths of time the towns continued their Old World way of life while partaking of the opportunities for freedom in the New World. The adaptations of the towns to the social changes of the eighteenth and nineteenth centuries in America, however, differed strikingly.

During the middle and latter part of the twentieth century each of the three towns has been losing population at a rate of 0.6 per cent a year.

The social order of Nazareth, the oldest of the three towns—established, financed, and guided by a handful of leaders—changed markedly within the first fifteen years of its founding as its financial base, the General Economy, collapsed and was replaced by private ownership and capitalism. As the leaders failed to keep pace with the changing social order in America, a second collapse was avoided only by opening the community to outsiders. Much of the old social order, including the class structure, was strong enough to survive, however, and the community continues as an orderly, quietly elegant place to live.

Bangor, organized a century after Nazareth, owed its founding to the entrepreneurship of the English and Welsh, who opened the community to other ethnic groups about forty years later, when laborers were needed to mine the newly discovered slate deposits. Bangor grew and prospered as its economy expanded, thanks to the construction of railroads and the opening of new markets for slate. The leadership of Bangor was as tightly controlled as that of Nazareth, although the basic philosophies of the two towns differed widely. Nazareth started as a communal society to benefit all equally, while the aim of the owners of industry and business in Bangor was to expand their individual power and financial control. Bangor had a longer initial period of economic growth and prosperity than Nazareth, but, unlike Nazareth, Bangor lacked community spirit and did not mobilize as a community to readjust to economic change.

Roseto, founded and developed in response to the custom of ethnic exclusion in the New World, has emerged as the most economically successful of the three towns. The Italians, like the Moravians, had strong community spirit. While seeking education, financial success, and identity as Americans, Rosetans retained their religious values and close-knit family structure and kept their community ethnically cohesive, rebuffing "infiltration" by non-Italians. Recently, however, as more young people are educated and with greater material prosperity, the value system of the Roseto community has begun to change. Attainment of the financial independence so earnestly sought by earlier generations has begun to erode the values that kept them distinctively Italian.

5
Roseto in Social Transition

As mentioned in Chapter 3, signs of impending social change were evident in Roseto as early as 1963. We predicted at that time that further changes, with perhaps a radical abandonment of Old World values and erosion of traditions, would be accompanied by a rise in the heretofore low death rate from myocardial infarction. Furthermore, we hoped to identify what aspect or aspects of the Rosetan society had contributed to their relative immunity from fatal myocardial infarction.

In 1966 we mounted a systematic sociologic survey aimed at sensing the winds of change and describing the values, attitudes, and behaviors that were emerging.

Of the 1,040 Rosetans over the age of twenty-one in

1966, 898, or 86 per cent were successfully interviewed in a house-to-house sociological survey that provided a comprehensive and detailed picture of the sociological characteristics of contemporary Roseto and enriched available demographic and statistical data. Comparing the findings with the earlier, less-extensive data we obtained as we observed and interacted with the people over a period of years as outsides, we were able to perceive the many subtle changes occurring in the community's way of life.

The Changing Social and Economic Scene

At the time of the initial health survey in 1961 we were aware that many in Roseto, mainly blouse mill owners, were relatively affluent, but, as mentioned earlier, we were not able to identify them from their dress, speech, or manner. Nor did their houses betray evidences of affluence. Most houses were neatly arranged in rows with a front porch on the street side and a well-kept garden in the back yard. There appeared to be an unspoken social taboo against any display of wealth except through generous hospitality with food and drink. Toward the end of the decade of the 1960's, however, such social restraints seemed to weaken. Interethnic and interdenominational marriages became increasingly frequent. The birth rate began to decline, and local churches noted decreases in church attendance. Women became more concerned about their weight, and several joined Weight

Watchers. Men turned to new leisure activities that affluence provided, joining country clubs and initiating a local golf tournament. Some took expensive vacations, visiting Roseto, Italy, and other parts of Europe, went on cruises, or traveled to Las Vegas and fashionable resort areas in New Jersey.

The gradual abandonment of the old ways in Roseto and the impending decay of the Old World culture were evident in the emerging preoccupation with materialistic values that accompanied increased education and growing affluence. During the decade from 1966 to 1975 many Cadillacs and other expensive cars appeared on Roseto's streets, including a handful of Mercedes-Benzes and even a new Rolls Royce. Several expensive houses costing upwards of $100,000 were built in an area of Washington Township that had recently been annexed to Roseto.

Rosetans not only had established constructive relationships with their Bangor neighbors but also, through their economic prosperity, had become more and more influential in the affairs of the Bangor area, which no longer excluded but included Italians.

Rosetans now serve on the boards of directors of Bangor and other nearby banks; are members of the same social, civic and religious groups; have opportunities to be educated in the same schools; and have successful businesses in Bangor and elsewhere. In short, there is evidence of growing assimilation of Italians in the entire Bangor area. As one respondent said, "For years they [Rosetans] strove for identity,

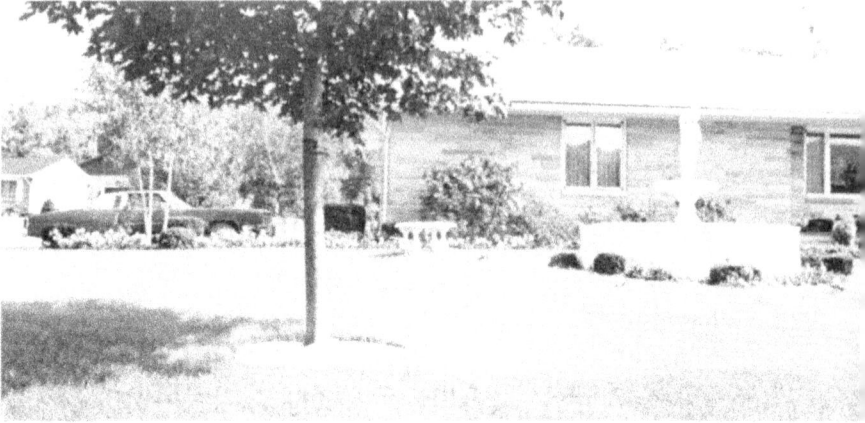

A new home and a private swimming pool in
Roseto—evidence of profound social change.

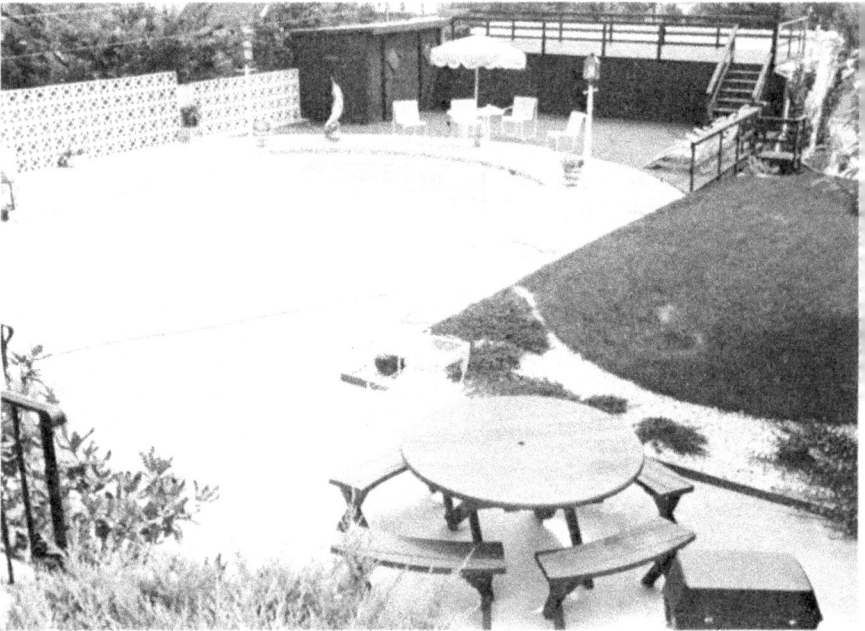

they were disenfranchised. Now they are in complete control. Their sons and daughters go to college and come home with professional degrees."

A striking development of the first half of the decade of the 1970's was the merger of the Roseto and Bangor Presbyterian churches. The English Presbyterians only a decade before had merged with the seventy-five-year-old Welsh Presbyterian church. The Welsh were aware that their ties and customs were rapidly disappearing from Bangor. The Welsh Song Festival has faced cancellation in the last few years, for few Welsh under the age of forty attended. The giving up of the Old Welsh Church was the relinquishment of one of the last remaining Welsh landmarks. The English and the Welsh were now confronted with their Italian Presbyterian neighbors, who had erased the barriers of language, lack of education, and Old World ways. The two churches finally merged in 1970 with a total membership of 530. The two ministers involved had tried to ignore the plan to merge the churches but ultimately were "pressured to retire." A committee composed of four members from each church was formed to accomplish the merger. They brought in a new minister, who was soon accused of being pro-Italian. The Roseto Presbyterian Church was put up for sale, but opposition grew in Bangor to selling the Old Welsh Presbyterian Church. Ultimately a "neutral" site for the construction of a united Presbyterian church was selected adjacent to both boroughs.

Studies of Other Italian Communities

In his study of Cornerville, a slum district inhabited by Italian immigrants and their children in the late 1930's, William F. Whyte observed that, as the American-born generation grew to maturity, the pattern of Cornerville life underwent many changes. The ties of community loyalty weakened, and the Italian families began to splinter as the younger generation asserted independence of its elders (45). In a related study of Italians in New Haven, I. L. Child described the feelings of "marginality" experienced by members of the second generation as they resolved the conflict of deciding whether to adhere to American or Italian ways (14). Pursuing the possibly deleterious effects of "marginality," Saxon Graham, in a study of chronic disease among various ethnic groups including Italians in Butler County, Pennsylvania, found that southern Europeans had initially lower rates of heart disease and hypertension than did ethnic groups from other areas of Europe and lower rates than those of the United States population as a whole. He noted, however, that with each subsequent generation in the United States the rates increased (20).

Francis A. J. Ianni, who studied an Italian community in Norristown, Pennsylvania, reported that by 1950 nearly 42 per cent of the Italian families had moved out of the colony (22). Indeed, in Roseto, when we first knew it, some second- and third-generation members of the community had moved away, while a few others were maintaining a marginal balance between Italian and American ways while living in Roseto. However, most Rosetans had chosen to remain in their Italian community in close proximity to family ties (3). As Luigi Barzini pointed out in his book *The Italians*, "the family extracts everybody's first loyalty" (1).

The Roseto Social Hierarchy

At the top of the status hierarchy as the social change evolved was a small elite group of wealthy blouse mill owners. They also derived income from other business ventures, such as textiles, slate, oil, and investments. These entrepreneurs, none of whom were college-educated, had risen to a position of economic power through hard work and ingenuity. They began to associate with other large blouse mill owners, slate-quarry owners, and professionals in surrounding towns through memberships in country clubs. Italian professionals living in Bangor or adjacent areas with relatives in Roseto were also high on the social scale because of their educational achievements.

Below this social stratum were the independent merchants and small blouse mill owners, primarily Rosetans between the ages of thirty and forty-five, some of whom were college-educated. Their attraction to status symbols—expensive clothes, large automobiles, and elaborate new homes furnished on the advice of interior decorators—reflected the beginning breakdown of former egalitarian standards among Rosetans. Most of the social activities of this group were carried on outside the community. This "fast-living group," as they were called by their neighbors, made periodic trips to expensive hotels in Atlantic City or to Las Vegas to gamble.

The skilled laborers, foremen, and others who were not business proprietors comprised the largest and most stable social stratum of the community. They continued to gather in the community clubs for their entertainment to drink beer, play cards, or just talk.

As a check on our findings, we attempted to identify the characteristics of the 14 per cent of Rosetan adults who for one reason or another were not interviewed in the sociological survey. They appeared to differ little from the group from which our information was obtained. Those who refused to be interviewed were slightly older than the subjects in our sample. They were generally less involved in community projects and activities. A very few of the oldest ones were unable to speak English. We were also interested in those interviewed who had not participated in the health survey described in Chapter 2. Their social characteristics differed in some interesting ways from those who did participate. Many of the latter were upwardly mobile, either educationally or occupationally, were employed in Roseto, and worked overtime on their jobs. A greater proportion of the nonparticipants, on the other hand, more than half of them men, were stable or downward-mobile educationally and occupationally, and fewer worked overtime. Also more of the nonparticipants were non-Italians. On the average they were about five years younger than the participants, had fewer children despite younger marriages, and were less involved in community and religious affairs than were the participants.

6
Myocardial Infarction in Sociological Perspective: the Sociology of Heart Attack

The social changes described in Chapter 5 began to be associated with an upturn in the death rate from myocardial infarction and the occurrence, for the first time in 1971, of infarction deaths in men under age fifty. Throughout the years of study of this community the indications were that the strength of unconditional interpersonal support and family and community cohesiveness had served to counteract the effects of life stress and thereby were a protection against fatal myocardial infarction. It was therefore of special interest to ascertain whether those who did succumb to myocardial infarction came from the mainstream of the Rosetan way of life and whether, because of the profound social changes or for other reasons, they found themselves relatively bereft of family and community support.

There is considerable precedent for the association of social deprivation or abandonment with sudden death. It is dealt with in descriptions of voodoo death and death from ostracism in many cultures (12, 50). In the United States sudden deaths are, by convention, attributed to myocardial infarction or to coronary arteriosclerosis. Such deaths in Western society, however, have been clearly associated with recent bereavement and with other forms of emotional drain (8, 33, 35, 48). Whether the antidote—emotional support—a characteristic of Roseto is important to the preservation of life itself becomes then the central question.

As background for the comparisons required, the nature of community support in Roseto and the price to be paid for it were examined. Although the effects of social change are buffered in an ethnically homogeneous and cohesive community such as Roseto, the price of being a part of such a community involves sharing common values and adhering to prevailing behavioral standards. Indeed, the maintenance of a high degree of community and family cohesion may require the social exclusion of individuals who are unwilling to conform.

Family loyalty under all circumstances is of first importance. Moreover, pride in family must carry over to the community so that a unified front is presented to the rest of the world. People must, therefore, work together, solving problems with resources inside the community insofar as possible. This process requires the maintenance of strong group sanctions, as well as alliances. Consequently, those who are unwilling to conform to the prevailing mores may be subjected to social exclusion. Thus membership in a highly integrated and close-knit community can involve responsibilities that may be taxing and burdensome.

Outsiders

Our interviews and questionnaires selected out a small segment of the population of Roseto who, according to the above considerations, could be classified as outsiders. They did not differ from the rest of the community in age, education, or religion but worked mainly outside Roseto and did not participate in Roseto social organizations.

There were three kinds of outsiders: non-Italians who married residents of Roseto and moved there, non-Italian marital pairs who had no ethnic or social ties with the community, and Roseto Italians who, despite their ethnic and social ties with the community, were excluded or excluded themselves by virtue of their style of life. Non-Italians, the true outsiders, rarely lived for long in Roseto. Roseto Italians with an uncharacteristic life-style, Italians who had moved to the community from elsewhere, and those with Italian spouses from elsewhere were usually marginal in Rosetan culture, even with respect to the location of their homes. Most lived on the extreme northern or southern boundaries of the community. These groups appeared to us to be at high risk for illness, especially myocardial infarction. When crises occurred, as they do before heart attacks, there was little or none of the family or community support so readily available to most Rosetans. Indeed, many marginal Rosetans seemed to have been seeking recognition and support through socially acceptable striving and occupational and financial achievement. If individual attempts at striving were thwarted or threatened, the individual might feel isolated and helpless and emerge a failure in the eyes of his peers. Similarly, if that individual and his fellow townspeople regarded each other as strangers, little or no community support was asked for or given. The organization of the individual's social life collapsed, and he was no longer a member of a group. A few who died suddenly of presumed myocardial infarction illustrated particularly well the importance of social conformity.

In Chapter 3 the classification among routine seekers, action seekers, middle-class mobiles, and the maladapted was described. Most of the action seekers and middle-class mobiles were young, primarily third-generation Rosetans. Since many of these had left the community or lived outside the mainstream of community life, there was little stimulus to the older second-generation routine seeker in Roseto to alter his way of life. Those mainly third-generation middle-class mobiles who continued to live in Roseto placed a very high value on education and sought to enhance their status. Interethnic and interreligious marriage was common among this group. Some of those who achieved a degree of affluence built fashionable homes on the outskirts of the town.

A few action seekers had begun to appear among Rosetans, mainly among the middle-class mobiles. They were considered the fast-living group by their neighbors. They entertained, traveled, and joined clubs outside the community in search of new experiences and opportunities. They placed the highest value on money. Many of these middle-class mobiles and action seekers actually identified themselves as outsiders in Roseto. Nevertheless, they continued to live there although maladapted to the social order. Most were beset by other stresses, especially marital discord. Our study found such individuals at high risk for the development of myocardial infarction as, by their life-style, they limited the family and community resources that could be available to them in times of crisis. The following two case histories are illustrative.

Case Histories

Born in New Jersey of Italian parentage, Mr. F was the eighth of ten children (six boys and four girls). His oldest brother, an alcoholic, had died at age fifty-six of a stroke. His father, a laborer born in Sicily, had died at age forty-nine of myocardial infarction. The mother suffered paroxysmal auricular tachycardia from the time of her husband's death and died at age seventy-eight.

Mr. F graduated from high school and wanted to go to college but lacked the financial backing to do so. At age twenty-four he married a Rosetan high-school graduate three years younger than he and moved to Roseto. Both he and his wife were Roman Catholic. They had two children, one son and one daughter. His wife worked as a sewing-machine operator, and he as a clerk typist. He held the same job for twenty-two years. He could type one hundred words a minute using only four fingers. His wife discouraged him from taking college courses because she felt it would entail too large a financial sacrifice. The marriage was marked by considerable discord over financial and other matters. Dissatisfied that he did not have a college education, he said that he wanted to make sure his son went to college. Two of his brothers had gone to college, paying their own way after their marriages.

"His whole life was under stress," said his brother. His wife was extravagant and unduly attached to her family, especially to her mother, with whom she spent a great deal of time. He was not happy living in Roseto although, according to his brother, "If he had had a happy home life, he would have been happy living in Roseto. His wife would harp at him like an old shrew." He often thought of leaving her but hesitated because of the children. After about ten years of marriage he began seeing other women. His brother said, "He wanted to enjoy life but was stymied."

He was not a member of any social or civic organizatons in Roseto and had no close friends. He was tense and self-conscious in the interview, stating, "I must have given you the dullest interview of all." He stuttered frequently, said that he had smoked two packages of cigarettes a day for most of his life and had drunk about twenty cups of coffee a day. He was not overweight and said he bowled for recreation. Although his brother and his family lived only a few blocks away in the same town, they had not seen each other except to wave in the two months before Mr. F's death. He said in an interview, five years before his death, "I don't fit in the town—I don't live like *they* do—I'm not like the Rosetans." When asked, in the same interview, whether he had been able to do what he wanted in life, he said, "No, I don't think I've accomplished it—that's why I'm nervous." He acknowledged being tense, nervous, and hot-tempered. He said he was not a practicing Catholic.

During the two months before his death he worked overtime on his job, and while his wife was convalescing from foot surgery, he also did the washing and ironing. Two days before his death, while paneling a room without help or power tools, he developed chest pain. The next day, while driving to work in nearby New Jersey, he began sweating profusely and experienced numbness in his arms and chest pain.

Shortly thereafter, in his doctor's office, he collapsed and died. He was forty-one years old.

Thus a man with a presumed genetic proclivity, because of his father's death from myocardial infarction at a young age, found himself out of the mainstream of Rosetan culture and died from a heart attack at a young age himself. The pattern was characteristic of other Rosetans who succumbed to myocardial infarction. Hard work and family and personal problems were common to most of them. In addition they emphasized self-reliance and responsibility for their own actions and hence enjoyed little or no family or community support in times of crisis.

The second illustrative case was that of Mr. A. He was born in Roseto, the oldest of four children, three brothers and one sister. In addition there were three half-brothers and five half-sisters from his mother's previous marriage. His father, a carpenter, had emigrated from Italy and had died at age seventy-two of aplastic anemia. His mother had diabetes and hypertension and died at sixty-four of myocardial infarction.

Mr. A. graduated from high school, worked as a carpenter, and at twenty-five married a German girl twenty years old, also a high-school graduate. He was Roman Catholic, and she converted to Catholicism. He described himself as a tense, nervous person who found it difficult to relax because, he said, "I feel I need to get things done and can't waste time."

Two years after the marriage Mr. A started his own

construction business in a town about twenty miles away. He worked overtime and smoked three packages of cigarettes a day for twenty years. Neither he nor his wife was a member of any of the social and civic organizations in Roseto. He had no really intimate friends in Roseto. The marriage yielded four children. His wife resented the amount of time his work kept him from home. Her interest was in family life. His was in making money. His mother died when he was twenty-eight. It was for him "the most unhappy time in my life. I tried to lose myself in work." He said he had thought about moving away from Roseto "to get closer to my business."

At age twenty-nine Mr. A was first hospitalized for chest pains when the construction business failed. After bankruptcy he founded a new company. This time the business succeeded financially, and Mr. A "lived like a king." He traveled to Puerto Rico, Las Vegas, gambled at the races, and bought expensive cars. He spent about a thousand dollars a week, gave wristwatches to his relatives' children, and responded generously to those who asked him for money or gifts without concern for repayment. He kept the problems of running the company to himself. His friend said: "You would never dream he had pressure on him unless you knew him. He always had it tough, but managed to get out of it." He enjoyed risk taking. Two months before his fatal heart attack, during a trip to Puerto Rico, he lost nine thousand dollars in one night of gambling.

He was admitted to the intensive-care unit of a local hospital for chest pains that started following his discovery that a bonding company had issued a fake bond in connection with a large contract. Upon being told that his EKG was normal, he signed himself out of the hospital against medical advice and engaged in a poker game until the early hours of the morning. During the two weeks following his hospitalization, he made ten business trips to adjoining towns in addition to resolving the bonding problem. The day of his death he got into a fistfight with a drunk, was arrested, and was required to post a one-thousand-dollar cash bail bond. Later that day he attended the wake of a friend in a nearby city and, upon returning home, collapsed and died. He was thirty-nine years old.

Testing a Prediction

In 1963, after two years of study in Roseto and neighboring communities, we predicted that, if and when Roseto's traditional close-knit, mutually supportive social structure began to crumble and traditional Old World values began to erode, the town's relative immunity to death from myocardial infarction would gradually come to an end. The original prediction was based on two underlying hypotheses: 1) social support from family and community is an important force tending to sustain health, and 2) those denied such traditional community support are at greater risk for myocardial infarction and sudden death.

Table 11 records the death rate from myocardial infarction per 100,000 men in each age group in Roseto and Bangor at each interval of our study from 1955 to 1975. The death rates for Bangor have remained within a comparatively narrow range, but in Roseto from 1966 forward there has been a striking increase in death rates from myocardial infarction, especially in the most recent five-year period, 1971 to 1975, when they reached the rate prevailing in Bangor. By 1965 evidences of loosening of family and community ties were clearly observable, and by 1970 materialistic and individualistic values had displaced much of the cohesive group concern of Roseto. This

TABLE 11

Death Rates from Myocardial Infarction for Men in Roseto and Bango
1955–75 (per 100,000)

Age	1955–61		1962–65		1966–70		1971–75	
	R	B	R	B	R	B	R	E
25–34	0	0	0	0	0	76	0	
35–44	0	35	0	224	0	0	352	1
45–54	139	288	0	435	204	606	220	2
55–64	0	1,106	357	1,111	556	800	1,140	1,0
Over 65	794	1,905	2,143	2,150	3,235	2,332	3,840	2,6

"Americanizing" trend with its erosion of established social values and traditions in the community of Roseto has continued, and with it there has been a significant increase in mortality from myocardial infarction, especially among men under fifty-five.

We were able to harvest some data among Rosetans suggestive of a basis for individual susceptibility to myocardial infarction and sudden death. From several individuals who died at age fifty-five or younger, statements recorded five to ten years earlier as part of our sociological surveys revealed evidence of breaking away or alienation from the traditional pattern of life in Roseto.

Table 12 records the death rates from all causes per 100,000 men and women in Roseto and Bangor during the period from 1971 to 1975. The data for myocardial infarction are similar to the figures for men in Table 11. Arteriosclerotic heart disease with failure remained less frequent as a cause of death in Roseto than in Bangor, but deaths over age forty-five from cerebrovascular accidents were somewhat more frequent in Roseto. Cancer as a cause of death also predominated to some extent in Roseto.

Other Studies

Other investigators have offered evidence of the healthful effect of emotional support, especially strong family and community structure. C. B. Thomas in a long-term prospective study of Johns

TABLE 12

Death Rates from all Causes for Men and Women in Roseto and Bangor, 1971–75
(per 100,000)

Age	Myocardial Infarction		Cancer		Cerebrovascular Accident		Emphysema Including Cor Pulmonale		HD with Failure Including Hypertension		Other*	
	R	B	R	B	R	B	R	B	R	B	R	B
Less than 24	0	0	0	0	0	0	0	0	0	0	72	37
25–34	0	0	0	0	0	0	0	0	0	0	0	50
35–44	161	50	80	81	0	50	0	0	0	50	36	100
45–54	160	136	80	507	160	34	0	0	0	0	36	68
55–64	440	707	880		440	67	0	34	0	101	440	169
65 and over	3,620	2,005	2,180	1,293	1,460	1,163	580	35	580	581	58	696

*Cirrhosis, renal failure, suicide, accidents, pneumonia, aneurysm, septicemia, brain tumor, etc.

Hopkins medical students found that the family values and relationships to which the students had been exposed as children could significantly predict subsequent coronary heart disease and other illnesses (38–40).

B. H. Kaplan and associates have marshaled evidence concerning the interaction between stressful circumstances and social support in the pathogenesis and prevention of several diseases (25). They recommend as preventive strategies deliberate efforts in child rearing to encourage affiliations and interdependence, emphasis on building morale with relationships among workers in industrial settings, and recognition of the potential value of strong religious commitments.

Susan Gore found, in a study of blue-collar men who had lost their jobs in company shutdowns, that a low degree of family support further exacerbated the stress of unemployment. Men who were unemployed and unsupported showed significant increases and variations in serum cholesterol, illness symptoms, and depression over unemployed men who enjoyed a high degree of family support (19a).

James Lynch has examined the question of human companionship in relation to health and longevity (29). He found that men and women living alone, especially if widowed or divorced, were at a significantly higher risk of early death. In his intriguing book he offers a persuasive argument for the healthful quality of human dialogue and love.

Victor Fuchs has called attention to the fact that two neighboring states, Nevada and Utah, are at opposite ends of the spectrum of mortality from myocardial infarction (18). The ethnic mix of the two states is very similar, both are among the nation's highest in level of education of the population, and the urban-rural mix is about the same in the two states. The average per capita income in Nevada is 15 to 20 per cent higher than that in Utah. For men and women between the ages of twenty-five and sixty-four, however, Nevada in 1960 had by far the highest death rate in the country. Utah had one of the lowest. Although the Mormon ban on drinking and smoking may be an important factor, Fuchs speculates that the stability of the social structure and the close family ties in Utah may play an important role in the discrepancy between the two states with respect to mortality from ischemic heart disease. Nevada's social structure is marked by fractured and disrupted family relationships.

Y. Scott Matsumoto has set forth a similar hypothesis to explain why Japan has enjoyed one of the lowest rates of coronary heart disease in the world (30a). Not only are family relationships extremely close and mutually supportive but the job situation is in sharp contrast to that in our country. Matsumoto describes the nature of the employer-employee relationship in Japan as a bilateral commitment. Being hired by a Japanese firm is like becoming a member of a family. Most employees are hired at young ages and remain with the same companies throughout their working lives.

The studies of Lot B. Page and associates may be pertinent as well. They reported physical examinations, blood-cholesterol and uric-acid measurements, and electrocardiograms on the native population of several of the Solomon Islands. They found no evidence of hypertension or coronary heart disease. They stated that, despite Western influence and adoption by some of Western diets and religious practices, "social and family roles had remained essentially unchanged" (32b).

John Cassel and his colleagues have found evidence that incongruity between a person's cultural norms,—that is, the attitudes and values that he grew up with—and the social setting in which he lives and works may contribute to ill health of many sorts, including ischemic heart disease (13a). Ischemic heart disease has begun to increase to an alarming degree in Yemenite Jews who have immigrated to Israel (11a) and in Ceylonese (32a). In both these populations social mores are changing rapidly, especially with regard to the emancipation of women and the acceptance of the materialistic values of Western culture.

It is very difficult to make rigorously verifiable inferences from observational as opposed to experimental data. For one thing, it is unlikely that on two occasions circumstances will be identical. That is hardly a reason to discourage such work, however. Shrewd observations have been the seeds of the growth and flowering of science on many occasions throughout history. Use of prediction to validate an inference from observations, a common practice among astronomers, was tried in the study reported in this book. It seems to be a useful strategy.

The data obtained over a span of twenty years in the Italian-American community of Roseto, when compared with those of neighboring communities, strongly suggest that cultural characteristics—the qualities of a social organization—affect in some way individual susceptibility to myocardial infarction and sudden death. The implication is that an emotionally supportive social environment is protective and that, by contrast, the absence of family and community support and the lack of a well-defined role in society are risk factors.

7
Summary
and Projections
for the Future

From a long prospective study of Roseto it seems possible to identify a social process pertinent to health. A group of proud, energetic, courageous, but poverty-stricken Italian villagers (*paesani*) came to live and work in the United States. They were forced by snobbish neighbors to look out entirely for themselves, to support one another for survival, and to form their own enclave. The family, traditionally the source of strength and buffer against adversity in Italian communities, played a vital role in enabling the Rosetans to cope with the early challenges and build a viable community. All the family members worked hard, and they worked for each other. As the years passed, their industry and enterprise were rewarded not only by economic success but also by the increasing respect of their neighbors.

From the beginning the sense of common purpose and the camaraderie among the Italians precluded ostentation or embarrassment to the less affluent, and the concern for neighbors ensured that no one was ever abandoned. This pattern of remarkable social cohesion, in which the family, as the hub and bulwark of life, provided a kind of security and insurance against any catastrophe, was associated with the striking absence of myocardial infarction and sudden death among those in the first five decades of life.

Now, nearly a hundred years later, a younger generation is less conscious of its heritage and less interested in preserving the unique character of its community.

During the past fifteen years the firm traditions and the secure ambience of Roseto have noticeably loosened, and for the first time young men are dying of myocardial infarction. Early evidences of the decay of the Rosetan culture followed its very success in coping with the broader American community. While the young people of Roseto were becoming educated through and beyond high school and even at graduate professional levels in greater numbers than were those from neighboring towns, few career opportunities were available to them in their small community or in the relatively economically depressed surrounding region of eastern Pennsylvania. When the young people moved away from their families, the first cleavage came in the traditional Rosetan culture.

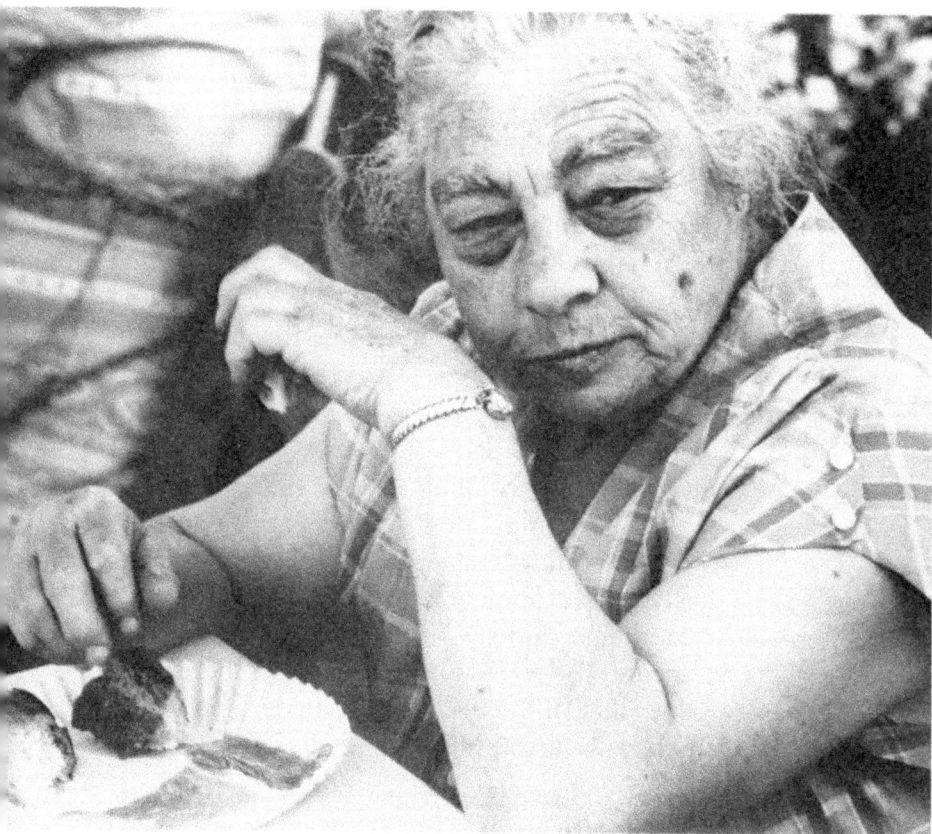

Refreshments at a birthday celebration in Roseto, 1962.

Other youthful and also middle-aged Rosetans contributed to the breakdown of tradition. As they were accepted more and more by their neighbors and became increasingly involved and influential in the affairs of the broader community, they acquired a taste for the materialistic rewards typical of the American dream. Nevertheless, for many years the more affluent Rosetans restrained their inclination toward material indulgence and maintained in their town the image of a relatively classless society. When a few began to display their wealth, however, many others followed. By 1965 families had begun to join country clubs, drive expensive automobiles, take luxury cruises, and make flights to Las Vegas. The rector of the Church of Our Lady of Mount Carmel noticed his congregation dwindling not so much because people were skipping church on Sunday as because they were attending fashionable churches in other localities. In 1965 opulent houses with broad green lawns, fountains, and swimming pools began springing up around the edges of town. By 1977 there were more than thirty of them. One housewife, after a year in such elegant surroundings, stated:

I'm sorry we moved. Everything is very modern here, very nice. I have everything I need, except people. When we lived in town, the neighbors were always in my kitchen or I was in theirs. We talked. We knew what was going on there and there was always someone around to help you and to keep you from feeling lonely. I miss that, but I guess I will never go back.

Social change and the fragmentation of families have been taking place in the Western world for centuries. It may be significant, however, that, as reported in Chapter 2, the lowest incidence of myocardial infarction is to be found in those parts of the

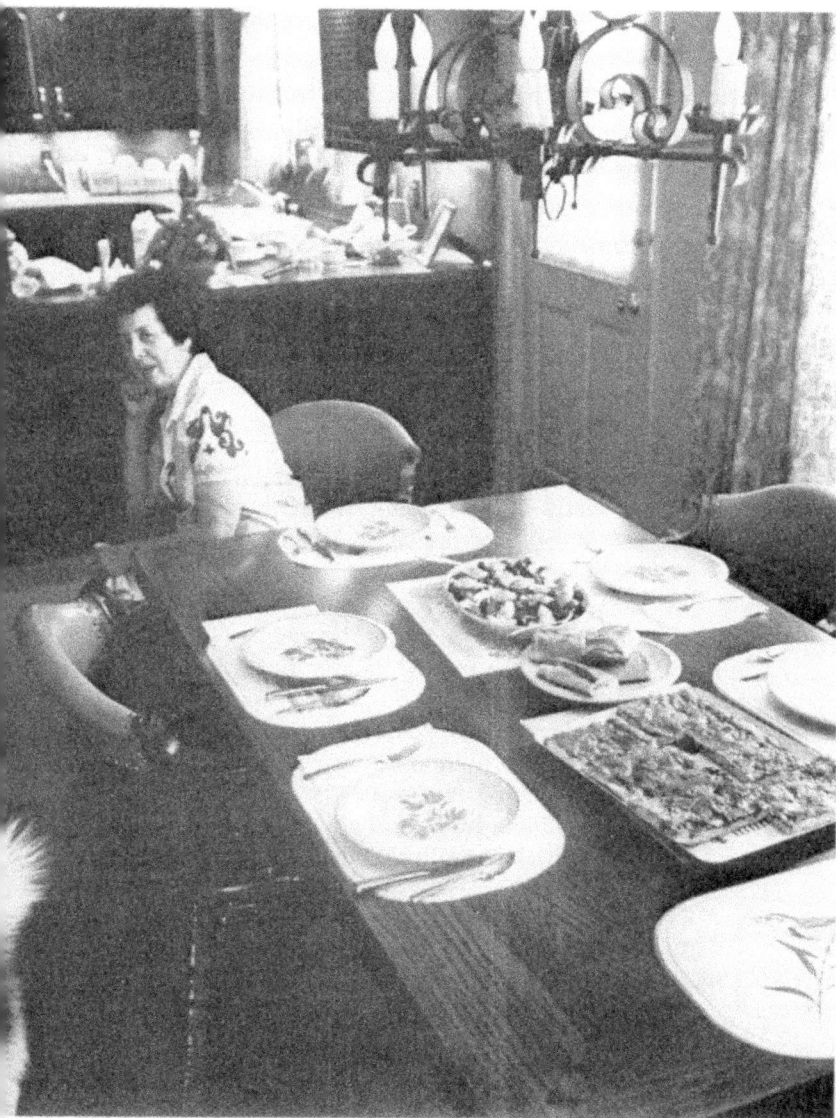

Refreshments in one of the new houses, 1971.

world where traditions of mutual interdependence and family ties are strong. Additionally it may be significant that sudden death is characteristically associated with rupture of human relationships and the emotional drain associated with bereavement, abandonment, or loss or misplacement in the scheme of things (8, 29, 33, 35).

The overwhelming impact of social exclusion was vividly perceived by William James:

> A man's social me is the recognition which he gets from his mates. We are not only gregarious animals, liking to be in sight of our fellows, but we have an innate propensity to get ourselves noticed, and noticed favorably, by our kind. No more fiendish punishment could be devised than one should be turned loose in society and remain absolutely unnoticed by all members thereof. If no one turned around when we entered, answered when we spoke, or minded what we did, but if every person we met "cut us dead," and acted as if we were non-existing things, a kind of rage and impotent despair would ere long well up in us, from which cruelest bodily tortures would be a relief; for these would make us feel that, however bad might be our plight, we had not sunk to such depth as to be unworthy of attention at all. [24]

In human beings the need for dependence on others has always been balanced by a drive toward independent self-assertion. The "now" generation of today calls loudly for demonstration of independence from parents and even from history. The result has been an increasing number of dropouts and of runaways—young people who are trying desperately to find their own identity independent of those about them.

The social disruption stemming from the loosening and fraying of close interpersonal ties may therefore be applauded as pursuing individuality, standing on one's own feet, being the master of one's own destiny. On the other hand, self-assertion and self-development may be fostered by education, a powerful shaper of attitudes and behavior in the modern world (23). As advanced educational and occupational opportunities entail greater participation in the outside world and wide social and cultural differences are created, individuals find that they share fewer common interests with other family members. Herbert J. Gans has pointed out that new occupational and educational attainments are likely to alter the structure of the Italian-American peer-group society (19). Rudolph Vecoli has observed that upward mobility among Italian Americans is usually accompanied by indifference toward traditional Italian culture and an accentuation of class social and cultural differences within the ethnic group (43). Clearly the process of class differentiation has begun among the third generation in Roseto.

The traditional atmosphere of Roseto encouraged interdependence and to some extent militated against the expression of individuality. Much satisfaction of social-emotional needs and social-emotional security derived, therefore, from conformity to community expectations. Being a part of the group, selfless to some extent, continues to be the price of acceptance as a good Rosetan, but with social change the sources of social and emotional security are becoming increasingly threatened. More Rosetans are working outside the town. Membership in local organizations has dwindled. The religious festival of Our Lady of Mount Carmel has become commercialized, and the religious processional that is the focus of the festival has changed. As late as 1965 a few of the women marched barefoot to express their humility and gratitude to the Virgin Mary for their many blessings in the New World. By 1970 there were no longer any barefoot marchers. Indeed, there were more spectators on the sidewalks than there were marchers on the street.

Roseto, Bangor, and Nazareth began with individually distinctive traditions and customs. Each adapted to the internal and external forces of change in different ways. Nazareth opened its doors to others, mainly those of German ancestry, but in the process did not completely lose its cultural distinctiveness. Bangor, on the other hand, no longer has a distinctive ethnic flavor. Roseto is at the crossroads determing its future course. Whether or not Roseto retains its ethnic exclusiveness, the character of the community will certainly continue to change. Middle-class material values and aspirations have already possessed some Rosetans and caused them to relinquish to some extent traditional values, remove themselves from the mainstream of the community,

and establish a new middle-class suburban development on the borough's western boundary.

The recent instances of myocardial infarction
among the young were found mainly among social
"deviants," those who to some extent had forfeited
community acceptance and support for material
"success." As the process of "Americanization" continues, as family and community ties continue to
weaken, and as Roseto's Old World Culture and traditional values continue to erode, we may expect increased numbers of fatal myocardial infarctions
among younger adults to the point where the epidemiological discrepancy between Roseto and its neighbors
may finally be lost.

Bibliography

1. Barzini, Luigi: *The Italians.* New York, Atheneum, 1964.
2. Basso, Ralph: *History of Roseto, Pa.: 1882–1952.* Easton, Tanzella Printing Company, 1952.
3. Bianco, Carla: *The Two Rosetos.* Bloomington, Indiana University Press, 1974.
4. Brindisi, Rocco: *Charities,* May, 1904, 443–504, col. 12.
5. Bruhn, J. G.: Sociological factors related to participation in a screening clinic for heart disease. *Soc. Sci. and Med.,* 3:85–93, 1969.
6. Bruhn, J. G., Brandt, E. N., Shackelford, M.: Incidence of treated mental illness in 3 Pennsylvania communities. *Am. J. Pub. Health,* 56:871–83, 1966.

7. Bruhn, J. G., Chandler, B., Miller, C., et al.: Social aspects of coronary heart disease in two adjacent, ethnically different communities. *Am. J. Pub. Health,* 56:1493–1506, 1966.

8. Bruhn, J. G., McCrady, K. E., duPlessis, A.: Evidence of "Emotional Drain" preceding death from myocardial infarction. *Psych. Digest,* 29:34–40, 1968.

9. Bruhn, J. G., Philips, B. U., Wolf, S.: Social readjustment and illness patterns: Comparisons between first, second and third generation Italian-Americans living in the same community. *J. Psychosom. Med.,* 16:387–94, 1972.

10. Bruhn, J. G., Wolf, S.: Studies reporting "low rates" of ischemic heart disease: A critical review. *Amer. J. Pub. Health,* 60(8):1477–95, 1970.

11. Bruhn, J. G., Wolf, S., Lynn, T. N., Bird, H. B., Chandler, B.: Social aspects of coronary heart disease in a Pennsylvania German community. *Soc. Sci. and Med.,* 2:201–12, 1968.

11a. Brunner, Daniel: personal communication, 1968.

12. Cannon, W. B.: Voodoo death. *Am. Anthropologist,* 44:169, 1942.

13. Carter, M. H.: One man and his town. *McClures Magazine,* 30:275–86, 1908.

13a. Cassel, John; Patrick, Ralph; Jenkins, David: Epidemiological analysis of the health implications of culture change: A conceptual model. *Ann. N.Y. Acad. Sci.,* 84:938, 1960.

14. Child, I. L.: *Italian or American, the Second Generation in Conflict.* New Haven, Yale University Press, 1953.
15. Epstein, Frederick H.: The Epidemiology of Coronary Heart Disease: A Review. *J. Chronic Diseases,* 18:747, 1965.
16. Facchiano, Monseigneur Annibale: *Roseto Valfortore.* S. Agata di Puglia, 1971.
17. Foerster, Robert F.: *The Italian Emigration of Our Times.* Cambridge, Harvard University Press, 1919.
18. Fuchs, Victor: *Who Shall Live?* New York, Basic Books, 1975.
19. Gans, Herbert J.: *The Urban Villagers.* Glencoe, Free Press, 1962.
19a. Gore, Susan: The effect of social support in moderating the health consequences of unemployment. *J. Hlth. and Soc. Beh.,* 19:157–65, 1978.
20. Graham, Saxon: Ethnic background and illness in a Pennsylvania County. *Social Problems,* 4:76–82, 1956.
21. Groover, M. E., Boone, L., Houk, P., Wolf, S.: Problems in the quantitation of dietary surveys. *J.A.M.A.* 201(1):8–10, 1967.
22. Ianni, Francis A. J.: *The Acculturation of the Italo-Americans of Norristown, Pennsylvania 1900–1950.* Unpublished doctoral dissertation, Pennsylvania State University, 1952.
23. Inkeles, Alex: Making men modern: on the causes and consequences of individual change in 6 developing countries. Am. As-

soc. of the Advancement of Science, Dallas, December, 1968.

24. James, William: *Principles of Psychology.* New York, Henry Holt and Company, 1918, 1:293.

25. Kaplan, B. H., Cassel, J. C., Gore, S.: Social support and health. *Medical Care,* 15(5):47–59, supplement, 1977.

26. Keys, A.: Arteriosclerotic heart disease in Roseto, Pennsylvania. *J.A.M.A.* 195:93–95, 1966.

27. Klees, Fredric: *The Pennsylvania Dutch.* New York, McMillan, 1955, 91–121.

28. Lord, Eliot; Trenor, John J. D.; Barrows, S. J.: *The Italian in America.* New York, B. F. Buck and Company, 1906, p. 39.

29. Lynch, James: *The Broken Heart: The Medical Consequences of Loneliness in America.* New York, Basic Books, 1977.

30. Lynn, T. N., Duncan, R., Naughton, J., et al.: Prevalence of evidence of prior myocardial infarction, hypertension, diabetes and obesity in three neighboring communities in Pennsylvania. *Amer. J. Med. Sci.,* 254:385–91, 1967.

30a. Matsumoto, Y. Scott: Social stress and coronary heart disease in Japan: A hypothesis. *The Milbank Memorial Fund Quarterly,* 48:9–36, 1970.

31. Musmanno, Michael A.: *The Story of the Italians in America.* New York, Doubleday and Company, 1965.

32. Nazareth Item Publishing Company: *History of*

Nazareth, Pennsylvania, 1740–1940. Nazareth, 1940.

32a. Obeyesekere, I.: Evaluation of risk factors in coronary heart disease in Ceylon. Paper presented at the Fourth Asian-Pacific Congress of Cardiology, Jerusalem and Tel-Aviv, September 1–7, 1968.

32b. Page, Lot B.; Damon, Albert; Moellering, Robert C.: Antecedents of cardiovascular disease in six Solomon Islands societies. *Circulation*, 49:1132–46, 1974.

33. Parkes, C. M.: Bereavement. *Brit. Med. J.*, 3:232, 1967.

34. Pisani, L. F.: *The Italian in America.* New York, Exposition Press, 1957, Chapter 9.

35. Rees, W. D., Lutkins, S. G.: Mortality of Bereavement. *Brit. Med. J.*, 4:13, 1967.

36. Scapellati, C. J.: *The History of the Roseto Presbyterian Church: 1886–1947.* Privately printed, 1947.

37. Stout, Clarke, Morrow, J., Brandt, E. N., Wolf, S. Unusually low incidence of death from myocardial infarction: Study of an Italian-American community in Pennsylvania. *J.A.M.A.*, 188:845, 1964.

38. Thomas, C. B.: Precursors of premature disease and death: the predictive potential of habits and family attitudes. *Ann. Int. Med.*, 85:653–58, 1976.

39. Thomas, C. B., Ross, D. C.: Precursors of hypertension and coronary disease among healthy medical students: discriminant func-

tion analysis. V. Family attitudes. *Jns. Hopkins Med. J.*, 123:283–96, 1968.

40. Thomas, C. B., Duszynoki, K. R.: Closeness to parents and the family constellation in a prospective study of 5 disease states: suicide, mental illness, malignant tumor, hypertension, and coronary heart disease. *Jns. Hopkins Med. J.*, 134:251–70, 1974.

41. *Transactions of the Moravian Historical Society.* Vol. 15. Bethlehem, Times Publishing Company, 1953.

42. Valletta, Clement: The Settlement of Roseto: World View and Promise. *The Ethnic Experience in Pennsylvania*, ed. John E. Bodnar. Lewisburg, Bucknell University Press, 1973.

43. Vecoli, Rudolph: The Italian-Americans. *The Center Magazine*, 7(4):36, 1974.

44. Ward, David: *Cities and Immigrants: A Geography of Change in Nineteenth Century America.* New York, Oxford University Press, 1971.

45. Whyte, William F.: *Streetcorner Society.* Chicago, University of Chicago Press, 1955.

46. Williams, Phyllis H.: *South Italian Folkways in Europe and America.* New Haven, Yale University Press, 1938.

47. Wolf, S.: Mortality from myocardial infarction in Roseto. *J.A.M.A.*, 195:142, 1966.

48. Wolf, S.: The End of the Rope: the role of the brain in cardiac death. *Canadian Med. Soc. J.*, 97(17):1022–25, 1967.

49. Wolf, S.: Psychosocial Forces in Myocardial Infarction and Sudden Death. Suppl. 4 to *Cir-*

culation, 40(5):74–83, November, 1969.

50. Wolf, S., Bird, R. M., Smith, J. J.: Personal Observations during W. W. II on New Guinea.

51. Wolf, S.; Grace, K. L., Bruhn, J. G., Stout, C.: Further data on death from myocardial infarction in Roseto, Pennsylvania and neighboring communities. *IRCS International Res. Comm. System*, 1973.

52. Wolf, S., Grace, K. L., Bruhn, J. G., Stout, C.: Roseto Revisited: Further data on the incidence of myocardial infarction in Roseto and neighboring Pennsylvania communities. *Trans. Am. Clin. & Clim. Assn.*, 85:100–108, 1974.

Index